Human Figure Drawings in Adolescence

By

MOLLIE S. SCHILDKROUT, M.D.

*Staff Psychiatrist, Long Island Jewish Medical Center
and Hillside Hospital*

I. RONALD SHENKER, M.D.

*Physician-in-Charge, Adolescent Service,
Long Island Jewish Medical Center
Clinical Assistant Professor of Pediatrics,
State University of New York, Downstate Medical Center*

and

MARSHA SONNENBLICK, M.S.

Staff Psychologist, Long Island Jewish Medical Center

BRUNNER/MAZEL *Publishers* • New York

SECOND PRINTING

Copyright © 1972 by M. SCHILDKROUT, I. R. SHENKER
and M. SONNENBLICK
Published by
BRUNNER/MAZEL, INC.
64 University Place
New York, N. Y. 10003

Library of Congress Catalog Card No. 76-183800
SBN 87630-050-6

MANUFACTURED IN THE UNITED STATES OF AMERICA

Preface

by LAURETTA BENDER, M.D.

Human Figure Drawings in Adolescence is a book that fills a real need. There are important publications on the drawings of children but nothing so comprehensive on the drawings of adolescents.

It has been prepared by a child psychiatrist, a pediatrician and a psychologist working in an adolescent service and clinic in a New York suburb. Significantly this is a medical and not a psychiatric service. Nevertheless, it was found that 50% to 60% suffered from emotional and personality problems often not indicated by their presenting complaint.

There is a review of the recognized uses of the drawings of the human figure by children. The authors utilized especially the works of Florence Goodenough, Karen Machover, and Elizabeth M. Koppitz. Goodenough established the use of children's human figure drawings as an index of intellectual development while she also recognized that the drawings revealed emotional maturity and, thus, psychopathology. Machover used psychoanalytic theory and the concept that the human figure drawing was a projection of the internalized body image in her psychodiagnostic interpretations of drawings. Koppitz preferred the interpersonal relationship theories of Harry Stack Sullivan while she determined maturational levels in children.

Adolescent patients (age 12 to 19 years), as an initial task on their first appearance at the clinic, were asked to draw a whole human figure and one of the opposite sex on separate sheets of paper. These were collected to a total of 1500 drawings. Drawings were also collected from inpatient adolescents, from a normal class of 6th graders (11 to 13 years) and a normal class of college freshmen (17 to 20 years).

In the preparation of this book, the drawings were studied without prior knowledge about the patients. They were evaluated and classified according to the chapter headings of the book and the clinical notes were added. A total of 192 drawings have been selected for the publication.

This method has evidently been successful with these authors. The book justifies very careful study by those who want to use human figure drawings in understanding adolescents. It is essential to learn the principles that are so beautifully described and illustrated here.

Without such careful study there needs to be warnings which the authors have suggested. Drawings alone cannot make a diagnosis. At the best, they suggest more intensive clinical studies of the patient, they "ring a bell," as the authors say, to call attention to a possible problem. No single test such as a drawing should ever be used alone for a diagnosis, or should be evaluated "blind" except in early stages of some research when insightful data is added subsequently. A full clinical study is always needed for a clinical diagnosis.

No human being can be exclusively classified into one of the categories described in the chapters of this book. Every adolescent will display some normal parameters, some kind of personality traits and his sexual preoccupations or level of sexual adjustment. Many from a clinical setting, where this material was collected, will also show neurotic traits, organic signs and some psychotic features and danger signs of acting-out aggressive impulses. One cannot expect that many drawings will show only one of these categories of features. Furthermore, subsequent events may show that such signs in some drawings were not significant of later pathology or acting-out.

Many drawings may not tell a clear story. These authors have used only something more than 10% of their collection. Many of the others may not have clearly demonstrated any features that could place them in any one category.

It should not be expected that a diagnosis could be made by matching an unknown adolescent's drawing with one in this book and accepting the same diagnosis for the new patient. A drawing is a piece of behavior. Although it is symbolic of the individual's total self at the time, no two individuals are alike in past history, social and intellectual maturity and personality adjustment. Thus even similar drawings may have different symbolic meaning.

However, the authors have rightly indicated that human figure drawings, especially when drawn at a time of crisis such as an adolescent presenting himself at a clinic for some kind of help, do show a level of maturity and reveal indications of emotional or organic deviations from the normal.

Follow-ups are always valuable. In human figure drawings they may show maturational trends or fixation of personality or pathological traits. They may help confirm the diagnosis. They may show the effects of treatment, especially with drugs. The authors have given us a chapter of follow-ups and scattered others of interest through the text.

Each chapter indicates a category of adolescent psychology and maturation, normal and abnormal. Each chapter and the conclusions are rich in concepts on the subjects covered, and concisely written. The book could be used as a text of adolescence and its disturbances in this culture and time.

Contents

ACKNOWLEDGMENTS

Without the aid and support of many, this book could not have been produced. The idea of including the drawing of the human figure as part of our routine evaluation of all clinic patients dates back several years. The usefulness of these drawings in the total evaluation of the patient soon became apparent to all team members. Their cooperation in obtaining the material and the discussions the material often engendered have, hopefully, been beneficial, in the final analysis, to our patients. We are grateful to these teenagers for their productions and for the interest they often expressed in their use.

A dedicated group of physicians and allied health workers through the years have made up the "Adolescent Clinic Team." They include the following to whom we give thanks for their help: Ruth Miller, M.D., Marie Louise Rie, M.D., Seymour Steinmetz, M.D., Stanley Blatt, M.D., Howard Scalletar, M.D., Vera Maitensky, M.D., Calvin Haber, M.D., Rita Faath, R.N., Ruth Sachs, R.N., Valentina Trops, M.S.W., Beatrice Eidinoff, M.S.W., Charles Wald, M.A. and Roslyn Nitkin, B.A. In addition, Anthony Musco, M.A. and Caroline Shenker, M.S. helped compile data.

We wish to recognize the support of the Department of Pediatrics of the Long Island Jewish Medical Center, Philip Lanzkowsky, M.D., Director, and Samuel Karelitz, M.D., Director Emeritus, whose efforts gave birth to our Adolescent Clinic in 1964. In addition, we have enjoyed the support and encouragement of the Department of Psychiatry, Samuel Lehrman, M.D., Director.

In the compilation of the material we would not have been able to succeed without the diligent aid of two medical students: Robert Yanover during the summer of 1970 and Jeffrey Good during the summer of 1971.

Finally we are indebted to Mrs. Evelyn Stoler for invaluable aid in typing and assembling the manuscript.

MOLLIE S. SCHILDKROUT, M.D.
I. RONALD SHENKER, M.D.
MARSHA SONNENBLICK, M.S.

CHAPTER I

Human Figure Drawings in Adolescence

INTRODUCTION

Man's need to communicate an affective human statement of himself as an object in space through the pictorial representation of his body requires no documentation. It exists all about us and always has, in myriad fascinating forms. What a man draws on paper or wall may be done as idle doodling or as a serious inspirational or studied task. Whatever its intent, it projects his mind's idiosyncratic image of himself or of his fantasied self. Through this image, the unconscious partially reveals itself. It is up to the observer to learn to read the message and to disentangle the cues in the human figure drawing, for surely it is a pregnant communication.

It is our purpose to study and to share with you the special significance of the human figure drawing during the turbulent years of adolescence. The work of others has firmly established the use of the human figure drawing as a developmental test of maturity and as an indicator of emotional and organic deviations from the normal, regardless of artistic training or native ability.

Interest in drawings as a means of obtaining clues to the personality, emotional status, and mental abilities of the artist has been developing for nearly one hundred years. Nineteenth-century studies dealt mainly with the artistic productions of institutionalized mental patients, or those of normal children. As early as 1876, Simon, in studying the art of severely disturbed individuals, observed relationships between features of the drawings and the symptom complex of the patient. Extensive investigations of "insane art" were undertaken by physicians in late nineteenth-century Europe. These studies addressed themselves to the use of art as a diagnostic tool and to the evaluation of the parallels between insanity and creativity, juvenile and primitive art. The height of interest in this area can be observed in the establishment of the Museum of Insane Art at the Heidelberg Psychiatric Clinic early in the twentieth century.

The study of children's drawings began as a part of the early child study movement, at its peak between 1895 and 1915. Investigators, frequently observing their own offspring or close relatives, collected numerous drawings over a period of at least a decade. Very early in the study of children's art, attempts were made to correlate drawings and mental ability. When Goodenough undertook her very extensive investigation of children's drawings in 1920, she was following less successful studies such as Schuyten's work. Schuyten evaluated the drawings of a large number of Belgian school children and established a "standard of excellence for each age." These standards were used as age norms so that drawings could be compared, and some impression of developmental level and intellectual ability established. Goodenough's text, *Measurement of Intelligence by Drawings*, published in 1926, encompassed age levels four through nine, and included 51 points of measurement by which the drawings could be judged. Her work is very well standardized and validated, and even today her "Draw a Man" test is still considered an invaluable aid in ascertaining children's intellectual level.

Although her test was not intended for use in evaluating children emotionally or in the diagnosis of psychopathology, Goodenough observed the possibility of utilizing analysis of drawing for these purposes. She felt that children draw from the world they know, rather than the world they see. In other words, a child, in drawing an object, projects his own experience, often altering external reality. Since drawings are so personally colored, Goodenough suggested that "drawings made by children might furnish considerable aid in the early diagnosis of personality disorders and mental maladjustments. From this statement one can observe a movement toward convergence of the two early paths of drawing analysis: psychodiagnosis and developmental child study.

Much interest has been maintained in drawing analysis as a projective technique. Many analysts and therapists working with children find drawings an invaluable aid. Anna Freud was one of the first child analysts to use drawings in her psychoanalytic work. Beginning in the 1930's Paul Schilder and Lauretta Bender wrote extensively about the art work of children in relation to diagnosis and therapy. Bender (1968) stresses the meaning of art productions as "creative activity, as projective phenomena and symbolism."

Many different drawing techniques have been developed to aid in diagnosis and treatment. Buck developed the House-Tree-Person Test as a means of exploring major areas of intellect and personality. Jolles' House-Tree-Person manual implements the use of this test by providing a detailed reference to a list of drawing features. Machover's study of human figure drawings is still considered a definitive text in projective analysis. This work, basing its interpretations on psychoanalytic theory, poses the basic premise that an individual drawing a person taps both consciously and unconsciously "his whole system of psychic value." The individual's internalized body image, evolving from a combination of his physical, physiological, psychic and interpersonal experiences, determines the features he selects in drawing a person.

Further work in drawing analysis is demonstrated in Hammer's text, *The Clinical Application of Projective Drawings*. Koppitz, somewhat dissatisfied with inconclusive results in applying Machover's work specifically to children, published a major text, *Psychological Evaluation of Children's Human Figure Drawings*. Her investigations use Harry Stack Sullivan's interpersonal relationship theory as a foundation, with the intention of exploring the child's developmental stage and his capacity for interpersonal relationships. She does not consider the "body image" hypothesis of Machover valid in her work with children and feels that the human figure drawing is not a portrait of the child's intrinsic lasting personality characteristics or his percept of his physical self. Rather, Koppitz feels that the drawing represents the child's current stage of mental development and his attitudes and concerns of the given moment, all of which will change in time due to maturation and experience. She offers well validated developmental norms, as well as "emotional indicators," signs which she feels reflect the child's anxieties, concerns and attitudes.

In his recent book, *Young Children and Their Drawings,* Di Leo pictorially traces the developmental evolution of children's drawings from their earliest scribbling through late childhood. A new technique is explored by Burns and Kaufman in their book, *Kinetic Family Drawings*. The child produces a "kinetic family drawing" in response to the instructions, "Draw a picture of everyone in your family, including you, doing something." It is felt by the authors that this technique offers a rich picture of how the child perceives the members of his family in relation to himself and daily life.

Our special focus is on the adolescent from 12 to 19 who presents himself for a wide variety of reasons to a medical clinic in a general hospital situated on the outskirts of New York City. The population represented is predominantly white, middle class. About 20% are from the lower socioeconomic strata and most of these are black. We serve patients between 12 and 19 with a relatively even age distribution except for a modest peak in the 14-year-old group. Almost half of these adolescents are referred by the guidance counsellors of the junior and senior high schools which they attend. Whenever possible, we maintain liaison with school and agency personnel for the benefit of our mutual patient. An understanding of the implications of the Human Figure Drawing could serve as a useful ancillary tool for trained guidance counsellors in selecting cases that require medical referral.

Early in our experience, it became apparent that 50% to 60% of our patients suffer from significant emotional or personality disorder. The presenting complaint in many instances has no obvious relevance to the psychopathology uncovered, since the clinic which provided the material for this study is not intended for patients with a known primary psychiatric disorder except in an occasional emergency situation. The clinic is staffed and directed by pediatricians assisted by two psychiatrists and a paramedical team consisting of a psychologist, social worker, nurse, nutritionist, residents and students. The high incidence of emotional problems in this relatively random group of adolescents seeking help has confronted our non-psychiatric staff with a challenging diagnostic burden. Since our goal has been to have one doctor treat the whole patient, avoiding whenever possible the fragmentation caused by excessive specialist referral, we have consistently searched for ways to intensify the psychological clinical acumen and sensitivity of the staff. In addition, economy of time is a realistic and important consideration. Hence, we have sought a device that might help to alert a variety of professionals working with adolescents to the existence of maturational deviations and denied emotional problems, as well as to indicate the degree of severity of existing psychopathology. The human figure drawing executed by the patient at the time of his first visit had proved its usefulness and validity in many previous studies of young children and adults. We decided to widen its use to an exclusive study of adolescents.

In collecting and studying about 1500 human figure drawings, our design has been a simple one. We have tried to avoid as far as possible the large number of variables which inevitably insert themselves into clinical psychological studies. At the time of his first visit to the clinic, prior to history taking and physical examination, we ask each patient to draw in pencil a *whole* person on a blank sheet of paper. He is then requested to draw a person of the opposite sex on another sheet of paper. The task is performed anywhere in the waiting room in an informal manner, unobserved directly by any member of the staff. No questions are asked and the drawings are collected by the clerical or nursing staff without comment. The drawings are kept separate from the charts and samples are selected as to their possible suitability for investigation of a number of problem areas. To widen the scope of our study, we added a collection of drawings done by a "normal" class of 6th graders, age 11 to 13, and a "normal" class of college freshmen, age 17 to 20. Another group of drawings was collected from adolescent in-patients admitted for acute medical or psychiatric conditions. Follow-up drawings were obtained after an interval of two to three years from some of the patients. Intelligence quotient of the patient is mentioned only when it has been formally established by psychometric testing.

In all instances we studied the drawings for indications of pathology or specific diagnostic indicators without any prior knowledge of the patient. We then turned to the case history, clinical findings, interviews and psychological test material (when available) for corroboration or negation of our working hypotheses of the adolescent's psychological difficulties. The pioneering work of Machover and the well documented studies of childhood drawings by Koppitz provided the major guideposts for our selection. Our goal has been to educate our staff to quickly recognize atypical features in these drawings and to follow these "smoke signals" with more sensitive and thorough interview and data-gathering techniques. In essence, the drawings serve as a device for case-finding. Our ultimate hope is to alleviate some of the emotional pain suffered by our young patients who, in many instances, will allow only that they have a surface complaint such as pimples, headaches, etc.

We focused our attention on the specific problems listed below, each to be treated in a separate chapter, in an attempt to determine the usefulness of the human figure drawings as a diagnostic tool in adolescence: the parameters of normalcy, personality traits, sexual identity, physical illness, organicity, neurosis, psychosis, danger signals (acting-out, suicide, homicide), and constancy through follow-up studies.

CHAPTER II

The Parameters of Normalcy

The word "normal" as it is used in this chapter is widely inclusive, signifying an absence of serious emotional pathology, intellectual deficit or personality malformations. Several areas are considered in evaluating the drawings, including variability in drawing skill. Cursory inspection of the work of a capable artist may lead to overevaluation of maturity level, whereas the converse is true in the production of the artistically untalented. If carefully appraised from a dynamic point of view, drawings of varying skill can give equally valid information about the emotional status of the individual.

Important in the assessment of drawings is familiarity with the stages of adolescent development, and the problems and changes to be expected at different ages. Blos divides adolescence into three major phases, beginning with early adolescence, ages 12 to 15. The dominant feature of this stage is an almost overpowering urge to return to dependency on the infantile mother image. The normal drive during this period is directed against this regressive tendency, and towards finding an object of affection outside of the family. Accompanying this effort to pull away from the parent is a weakening of the superego. The ego is thus left relatively defenseless, resulting in considerable struggle to maintain equilibrium against the onslaught of sexual and aggressive impulses. The dependency upon the parent is seen commonly in drawings of both boys and girls in the form of obvious midline emphasis, numerous buttons and belt buckles. Efforts to control impulses in the face of weakening superego and ego are reflected in the frequent use of stripes, plaids, dots and other designs covering much of the body. Concomitant with this is the use of body shading and emphasis in sexual regions, reflecting the anxiety experienced over the dramatic physical changes which are taking place. The girl normally goes through a stage of bisexuality, in which she feels she possesses the characteristics of boy and girl simultaneously. Psychoanalytic theory postulates that the female has greater difficulty in the resolution of the oedipal complex. In a considerable number of drawings by 13-year-old girls, the male is drawn first, or the drawing is sexually ambiguous and spontaneously labeled "tomboy," "boy-girl" or "neuter." Boys are more defended against awareness of their bisexuality and rarely draw female figures first. Further discussion of this aspect of development appears in Chapter IV on *Sexual Identity*.

Middle adolescence, beginning at 15, brings with it a very strong resurgence of oedipal feelings and the search for a love object of the opposite sex. The most important achievement during this period is the resolution of the oedipal conflict through identification with the parent of one's own sex, and the establishment of a feminine or masculine role. During this phase there is increased narcissism as compensation for the "loss" of the parent. Drawings may appear grandiose by depicting an idealized physical image. The 16-year-old girl may draw a seductive, fashionably dressed female while the boy may portray a male of obvious athletic prowess. Intellectualization used as a major defense during this time is reflected in items such as peace symbols, representing idealism, and in meticulous detailing. Through much of this stage, dependency conflicts and sexual identity confusion may persist. However, as middle adolescence approaches its close toward the eighteenth year, sexual identification difficulties tend to diminish.

Late adolescence is a time during which consolidation occurs within the ego. There is greater constancy in both sexual identification and object choice, and stabilization in the mechanisms of defense which protect the psychic integrity. Hopefully, the individual of 18 or 19 approaches maturity with some feelings of equanimity, self-esteem and purpose. Drawings of the late adolescent should be relatively free of earlier anxiety indicators such as shading and overworked lines, possess obvious differentiation between male and female in body contours, and convey a feeling of adequate integration. Thus, in the normal adolescent, one sees a marked developmental evolution in the drawings done between ages 12 and 19.

Cultural factors idiosyncratic to youth have a decisive influence on figure drawings. Clothing, makeup and hairstyle are a reflection of fashion specifically designed for the young. Many of the normal drawings show the unisex appearance currently in vogue. Recently the drawings of black adolescents have shown Afro haircuts and other symbols which reflect growing black identity.

The absence of serious pathological features in a drawing is necessary before it can be considered within the normal range. Obvious lag in development, such as the appearance of strong dependency signs or ambiguity in sexual identification in a 19-year-old's drawings is indicative of difficulties. Disproportionately large or small figures, absence of hands, feet, arms, face, etc., shaky or broken lines, poor integration of body parts or lack of appropriate demarcations are all significant of some type of disturbance. Bizarreness, inclusion of details which are unusual or highly idiosyncratic, and obvious transparencies do not appear in normal drawings. Most important of all in the evaluation of normalcy in drawings is the total qualitative aspect or Gestalt. A drawing conveys an affective as well as a cerebral communication to which the observer makes a total response before analyzing the details.

FIGURE 1

F.A.   Age 12   Female

This girl is an average student and presents no obvious emotional or behavioral difficulty.

Drawing: Artistic ability is of mediocre quality yet the drawing is adequately proportioned and integrated. The heavy lines outlining body, arms and legs, and the rather rigid posture reflect the need to control newly emerging feelings and impulses. Concomitantly, an elaborate design over the clothing is used defensively. Dependency and midline emphasis, typical of this age, appear in the form of a star in the middle of the chest. The drawing shows little sexual differentiation in its absence of feminine body contours.

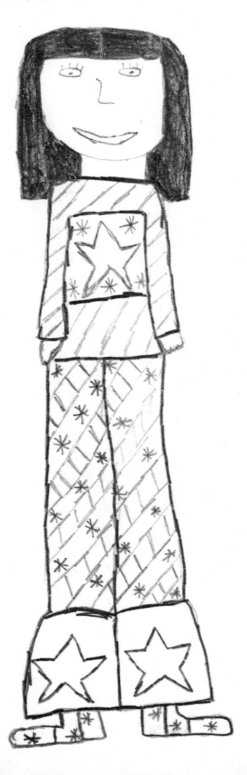

FIGURE 1   9

FIGURE 2

This boy is an average student with a good social adjustment.

Drawing: The features which make this drawing typical for youngsters of this age are buttons, and shading over the upper body and foot area. Masculinity is stated more obviously in 13-year-old boys' drawings than femininity is in the drawings of girls of the same age. The beard, mustache and cigarette are rather typical symbols depicting the desired manhood.

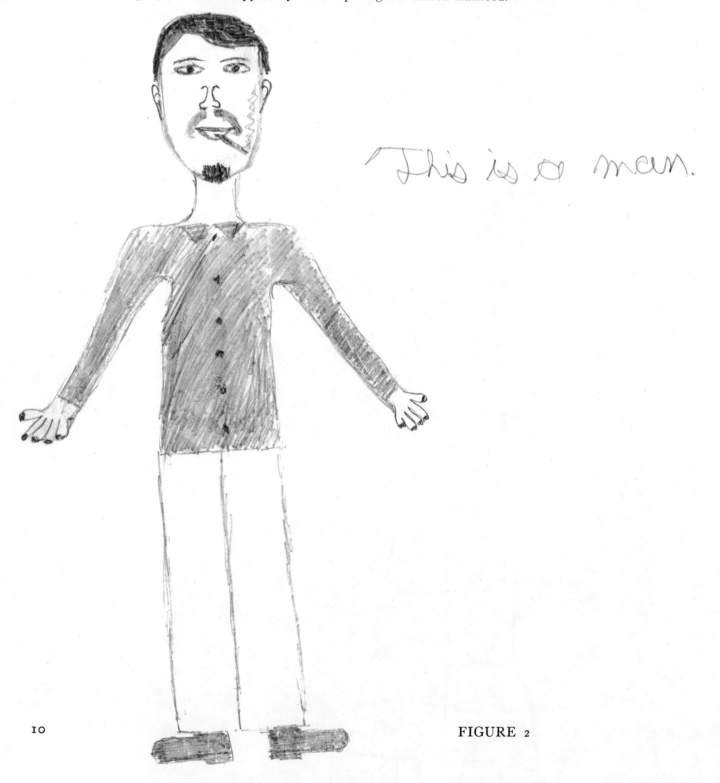

This is a man.

FIGURE 3

F.C.   *Age 13*   *Female*

Black girl of superior intelligence.

Drawing: Artistic ability and good intellectual endowment are evident in the drawing. Many features, including the drawing of a male figure first, are common to this stage. Noteworthy are the Negroid features and Afro hair style which are indicative of the girl's need to find a black identity.

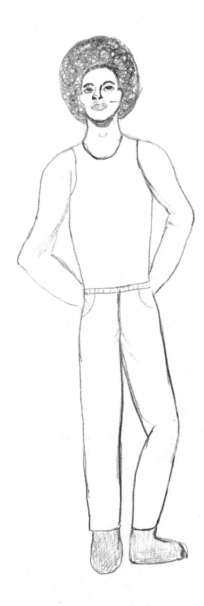

FIGURE 3

FIGURE 4

F.D.   *Age 12*   *Female*

This girl is a well adjusted black youngster.

Drawing: The unusual feature in this drawing is the heavy shading through-out the face and body area. Such shading is a relatively rare feature in black adolescent drawings. Identity is more commonly expressed in facial features and hair style.

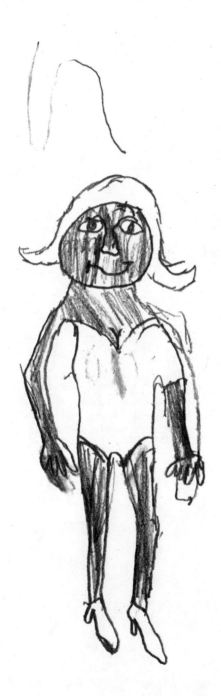

FIGURE 4

FIGURE 5

F.E.   *Age 13*   *Female*

This girl is an average student with adequate social adjustment.

Drawing: Possessing most features typical for this stage, this figure was designated spontaneously as "neuter." Several drawings in the series had similar designations and illustrate the bisexuality of the early adolescent girl.

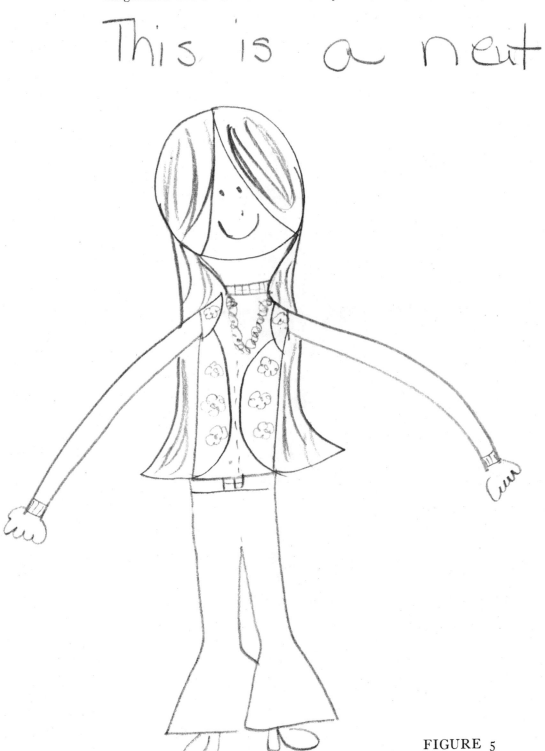

FIGURE 5

FIGURE 6

F.F.　　　　　*Age 15*　　　　　*Male*

This boy has a good social and school adjustment. He is an excellent guitar player and leads his own band.

Drawing: The shading and sketchy line quality indicate anxieties common in middle adolescence. The dress, hair style and beard are emblems of identification with the culture. The guitar serves several functions, in that it ensures a place in the culture and an assertion of individual ability and worth. It is a badge of adequacy which helps to shield the person, uncertain at this age, from standing alone and exposed.

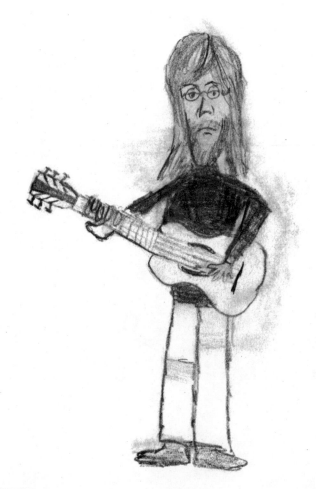

FIGURE 6

FIGURE 7

F.G.   *Age 15*   *Female, high school student*

This girl is very sociable, well accepted by peers and academically successful.

Drawing: The drawing is well integrated. Attempts at controlling impulses are suggested in the ribbing at neck and waist, and in the pendant. Hairdo is stylish and somewhat seductive. The heavier line pressure in the foot area, and the lines and ties on the shoe reflect the ambivalence about stepping out on her own, a common conflict at this stage. The total quality of the drawing is of a relatively emotionally healthy youngster experiencing the problems typical of middle adolescence.

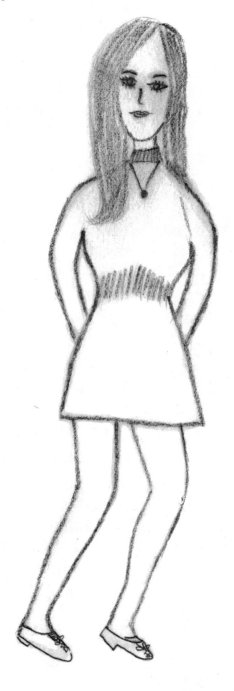

FIGURE 7   15

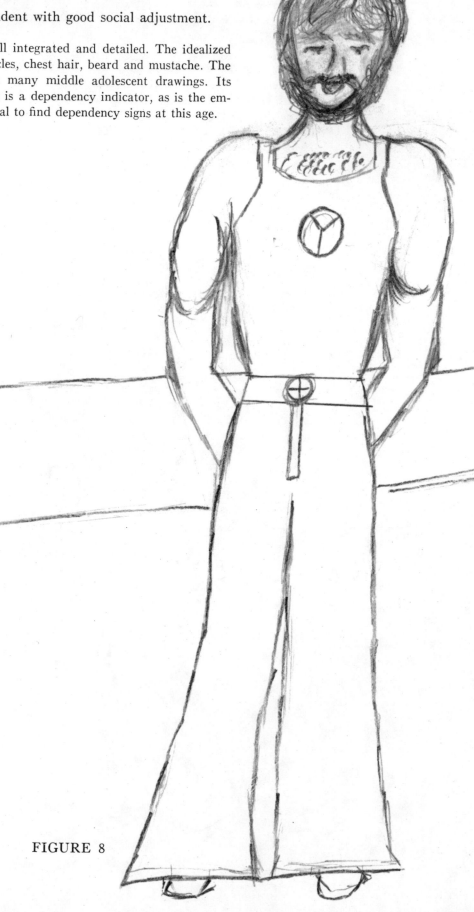

FIGURE 8

F.H.   *Age 16*   *Male*

This boy is a high school student with good social adjustment.

Drawings: The human figure is well integrated and detailed. The idealized male is presented with bulging muscles, chest hair, beard and mustache. The peace symbol appears currently in many middle adolescent drawings. Its placement in the center of the chest is a dependency indicator, as is the emphasized belt buckle. It is not unusual to find dependency signs at this age.

FIGURE 9

F.I. *Age 15* *Female*

The girl is a good student, somewhat shy with peers.

Drawing: This figure is an idealized female, with perfect feminine figure and very stylish dress. The rather stiff posture and compulsive striping of the neck and leg are efforts to control fantasies and impulses. Midline emphasis is still very common at this age, as dependence versus independence is a major developmental issue.

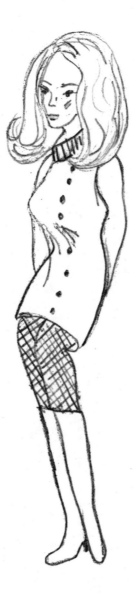

FIGURE 9

FIGURE 10

F.J.   *Age 17*   *Female*

Adequate social adjustment.

Drawing: The figure is well proportioned and much of the compulsive detailing common in earlier drawings has disappeared. Line quality is somewhat sketchy, but the drawing gives the impression of being well put together.

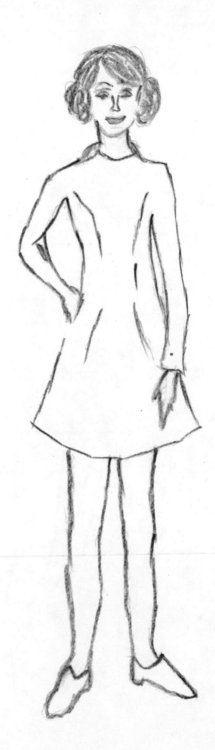

FIGURE 10

FIGURE 11

F.K.   *Age 19*   *Female*

Unknown college student.

Drawing: The figure is definitely feminine although body contours, such as the bustline, are not clearly delineated. There is still some difficulty with control of body impulses, as evidenced in the horizontal striping. The shaded legs and feet express concern over direction and standing on her own. The total quality of the drawing is age appropriate to a late adolescent girl. In many of the normal drawings evidence of incomplete resolution of conflicts of earlier stages still exist.

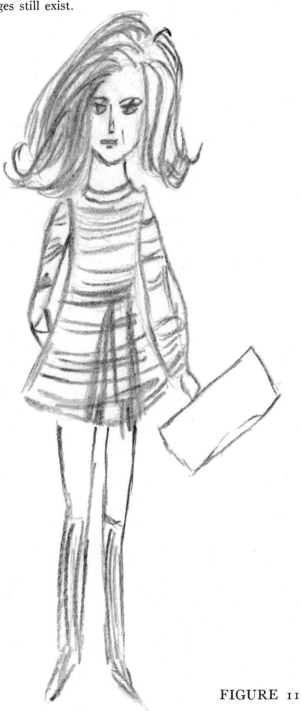

FIGURE 11

FIGURE 12

F.L.   *Age 19*   *Female*

Unknown college student.

Drawing: The drawing is very well proportioned and glamorous in appearance. Line quality is good and dependency and anxiety signs are not present.

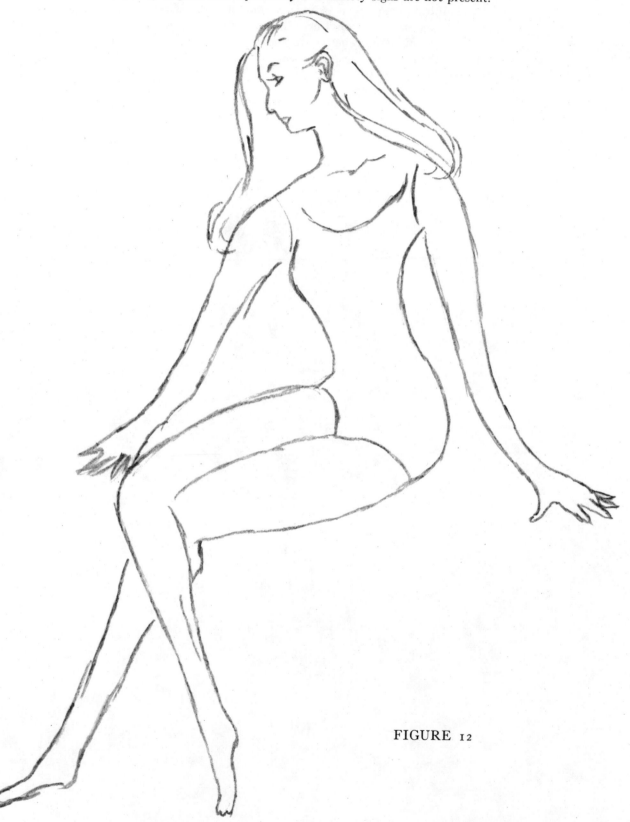

FIGURE 12

FIGURE 13

F.M.   Age 19   Male

College student. He is very outgoing and academically successful.

Drawing: The drawing, although not artistically talented, is well integrated and gives the impression of a fair degree of strength and sense of masculinity. Some earlier conflicts are still present as indicated in the striped shirt, sketchy line quality and hidden hands. The total quality of the drawing places it within the normal range.

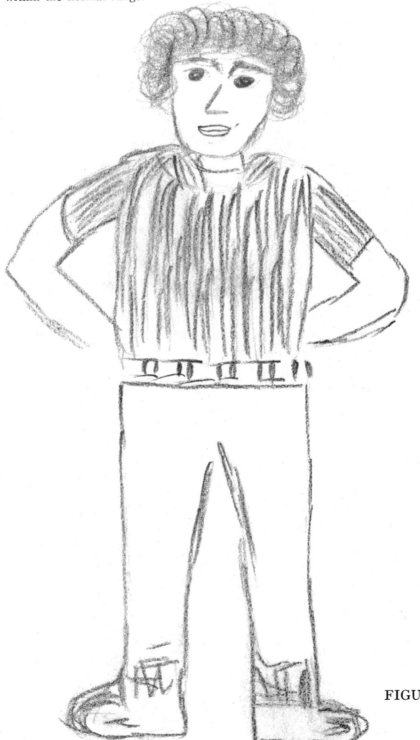

FIGURE 13

CHAPTER III

Personality Traits

The study of many hundreds of human figure drawings done by a random selection of adolescents leads us to the conclusion that it is not possible in most instances to pinpoint a personality disorder diagnosis from our samples. It is, however, not difficult to find evidence of specific traits that leads one to investigate further through examination of the history, interview and psychological testing when needed. The "Diagnostic and Statistical Manual of Mental Disorders" formulated by the American Psychiatric Association (1968) lists fifteen major types of personality disorders and defines them as follows: "This group of disorders is characterized by deeply ingrained maladaptive patterns of behavior that are perceptibly different in quality from psychotic and neurotic symptoms. Generally, these are lifelong patterns, often recognizable by the time of adolescence or earlier."

We have been impressed by the large number of drawings that clearly demonstrate an adolescent's image of himself as immature and inadequate. These are drawings that do not show the bizarre qualities of psychosis or the specific anatomical distortions seen in the organically impaired. They are quite simply the portraits of younger children. They do not represent a physical mirror image of a youth, sometimes as old as 18, but rather a psychic inner image reenforced by years of feedback from the significant others in his life who have continued to perceive him as a young child. Specific qualities which appear in certain drawings suggest that we may be dealing with paranoid, schizoid, compulsive, hysterical, passive or antisocial personality development. In the following pages we shall present illustrations of these deviations from the normal with a brief clinical history and impression.

FIGURE 14

G.B.   *Age 17*   *Female*

The patient has long been unhappy at home, feeling that her brothers are preferred by her parents. A year ago she suffered a drug psychosis from LSD and hashish for which she was hospitalized. Drug abuse has now been replaced by food abuse, resulting in obesity.

Drawing: The girl is a fully developed but dependent puppet, with incomplete feet to stand on. Details of clothing are omitted, implying feelings of emptiness and restricted imagination. The outstretched arms and fingerless hands appear to be waiting to be manipulated by some outside force. The rippled skirt hem and legs held close together point to sexual anxiety, perhaps stimulated by fantasies about her brothers towards whom she expresses so much rage. It is clear that she does not feel in control of her own impulses.

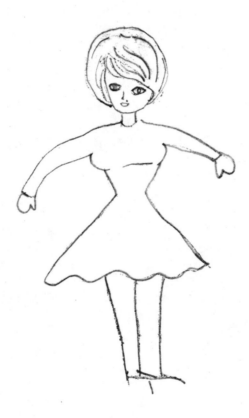

FIGURE 14

G.A.   *Age 16*   *Female*   *Average I.Q.*

The patient has always had learning problems, lack of self-confidence and lack of friends. As a young child she showed great separation anxiety and has continued to cling tenaciously to her mother. She bitterly resents her younger sister. She dresses immaturely, whines and complains constantly. Psychotherapy has helped to make her a little more outspoken, but she has resisted change and maturation through strong passive resistance.

Drawings: Anatomical details are correct and present in figs. 15 and 16, but are crude and infantile in quality. This is especially manifest in the short outstretched arms with jagged tooth-like fingers. Such hands are obviously ineffectual, but can get a claw-like grasp on objects. The clothing details are compulsive. The broad stance gives more support, but the feet are going in opposite directions.

A year later the patient draws figure 17, labeled "boy," that shows further deterioration. Compulsivity has further restricted her imagination, as shown by the monotonously striped clothing. Feet are omitted, making the figure still more powerless to move.

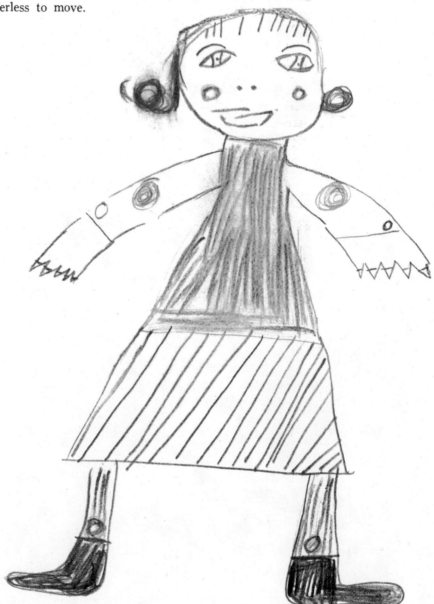

FIGURE 15

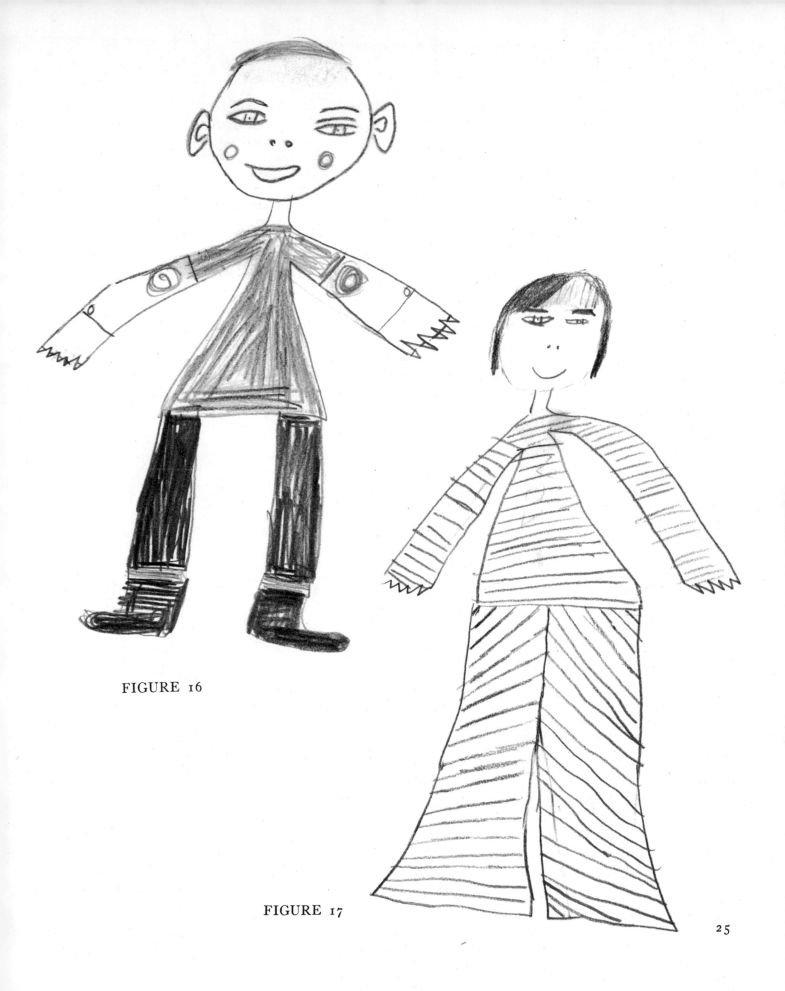

FIGURE 16

FIGURE 17

25

G.C.   *Age 14*   *Male*   *Average I.Q.*

The patient was referred for study of short stature and chronic school problems. In school he is immature, inattentive and silly. At home he is childishly demanding, becoming abusive when not gratified. He is hostile toward his siblings and prefers the company of younger children. His father died when the patient was 4 months old and he no doubt suffered severe emotional deprivation.

Electroencephalogram is negative and no evidence of organicity could be established.

Drawings: They are immature, robot-like, bland. Squared shoulders with poorly placed spindle arms and hidden hands imply feelings of being ineffectual and having something to hide. The only differentiation between the sexes is the curly hair of the female and the emphasis on her eyelashes. The peculiar oval space between the legs of both drawings further underscores his unconscious questioning of what constitutes maleness. The figures are poised on a scribbled base, indicating the need for support. These drawings have an "organic" quality, demonstrating the close link between a developmental maturational lag of genetic origin and that caused by emotional deprivation and humiliation.

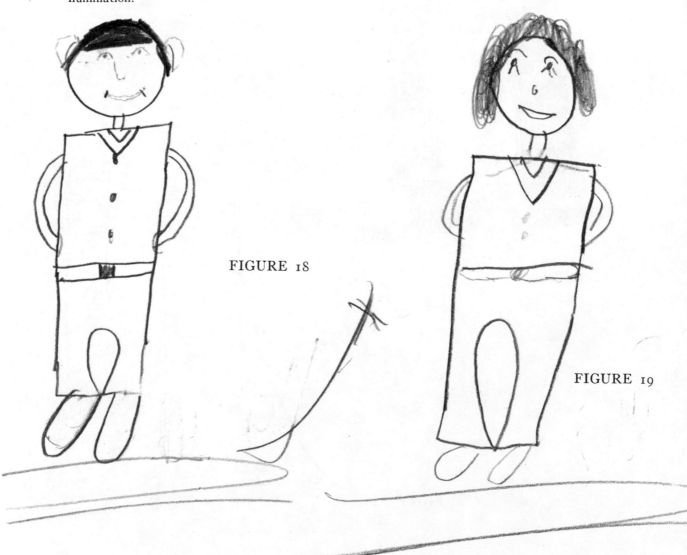

FIGURE 18

FIGURE 19

G.D.   *Age 18*   *Male*

The patient came to the clinic because of acne and pain in the knee when walking. His parents are divorced. He dislikes his father for having disappointed him and is very close to his mother. He does not work hard in school and actually dropped out for a while, losing a term.

Drawings: The male is an accurate self-representation. He passively sits and waits, hands folded. There is a suggestion of anxiety in the shaded line quality.

The female actively reaches out, probably a wish-fantasy involving his mother and other women.

The history and the drawings tell the same story: passive-dependent personality.

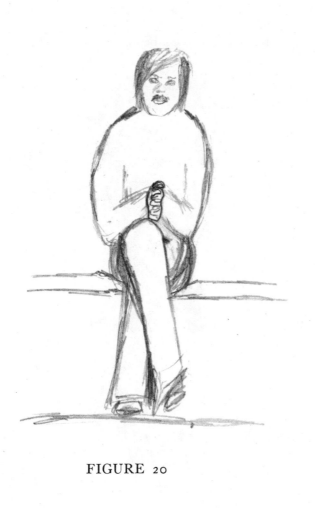

FIGURE 20

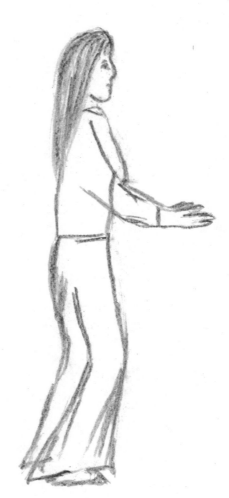

27

FIGURE 21

G.E.   *Age 13*   *Male*   *Average Intelligence*

The patient is dyslexic and attends a special class. He is somewhat immature, superficially compliant and unable to talk about his learning problem.

Drawings: The boy is silly, a stupid looking clown. His crossed eyes cannot see straight, therefore cannot read. Crossed eyes also imply covert hostility, hence the common expression, "I was so mad, I couldn't see straight." The huge incisor teeth in the wide mouth are intended to convey feelings of stupidity, but also show veiled hostility. The conventional neat clothing, including a tie, emphasizes his outward compliance. The inclusion of a tie on a 13-year-old also indicates phallic concern, as do the shaded trousers, crossed legs and protective hand. The other hand leans on a desk (the teacher's?), while the floor is drawn for further support of his dependency needs. The female looks angry, baring a mouthful of teeth. She also has crossed eyes, a phallic nose, one arm going into the body with an outwardly displaced thumb. The raised arm seems to be signaling "stop." The legs are awkwardly sloped outwards. Some of these anatomical errors may be due to his perceptual difficulties.

FIGURE 22

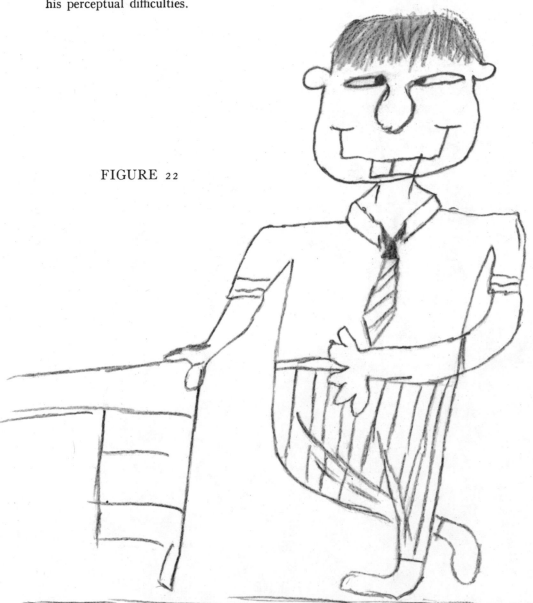

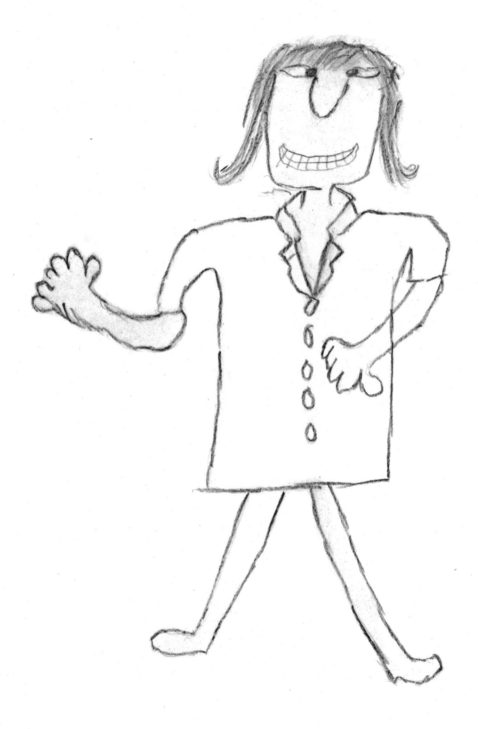

FIGURE 23

G.F.   *Age 16*   *Male*   *Average Intelligence*

The patient came to the clinic to "please" his mother. He has been a chronic underachiever and a drug abuser, chiefly taking barbiturates and amphetamines. His manner is soft and bland, belied by the presence of a facial tic. He complains of boredom, has no goals, no opinions and no commitments. An undercurrent of depression and anxiety is palpable.

Drawings: They demonstrate his feelings of emptiness through blindness (no pupils) and lack of detail. A single horizontal line at the waist indicates that the male is wearing trousers. The girl, who has a poorly proportioned figure, is nude but lacks distinguishing female anatomical characteristics. The unattractive hairless male lacks power and virility. His head, separated from his body by a long thin neck, looks pinned on and incapable of controlling his impulses. Teeth reveal his oral aggression. The petal fingers, only four on the left hand of the girl, are a sign of immaturity.

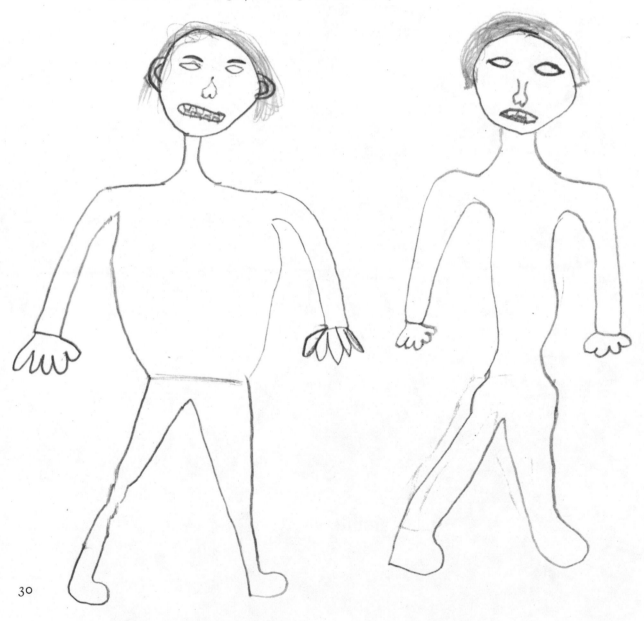

30

FIGURE 24   FIGURE 25

G.G.   *Ages 13½ & 16*   *Male*

The patient came to the clinic because of lower back pain and was found to have epiphysitis of the spine. His parents are separated. His mother described him as stubborn and argumentative, tenacious in his wish to be "always right." He expressed ambivalent feelings towards both parents. He is an excellent student, highly goal directed, but unpopular with his peers.

Drawings: At 13 he drew a faintly outlined male figure lacking facial features, hands and feet. It suggests a schizoid adaptation. The open mouth in profile is present but barely visible. He refused to draw a girl. Anxiety and withdrawal are evident.

At 16 he drew a male in profile with a strong pencil line, compulsively striping the shirt and anxiously shading the pants with scribbled lines. The figure is slanted backwards and stands on a base line, indicating feelings of insecurity. The arm is either foreshortened or hidden in a pocket. Most interesting is the jutting wide open mouth which appears to be arguing or yelling, a prominent activity of the patient. The nose is phallic, the eye almost closed.

The female figure, done willingly at age 16 in contrast to his earlier refusal, is a much smaller doll-like frontal figure. She is pleasant, cute, insignificant. Breasts are indicated.

The patient is now more sure of himself, but still hostile and aloof in personality.

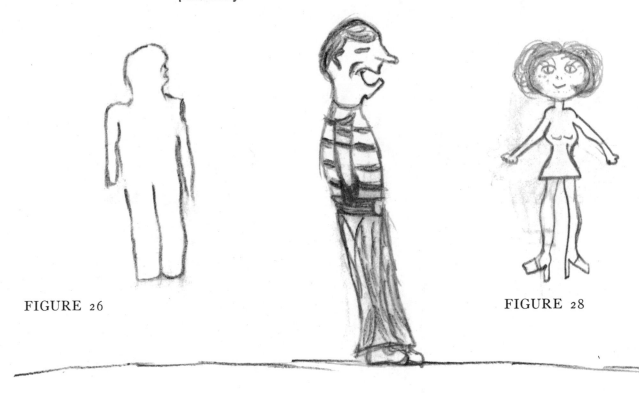

FIGURE 26

FIGURE 28

FIGURE 27

G.H.   *Age 16*   *Female*

The patient is overweight, always tired and sluggish. She came to the clinic apprehensive about blood tests, fearing that blood would be taken from her knee. Her general manner is immature.

Drawings: The wide-eyed stare of both figures is typically hysterical in character. Hands placed in the pockets or behind the back indicate guilt and an attempt to control "forbidden" impulses. The legs are amputated, thus eliminating the part of the body she fears will be hurt by a needle.

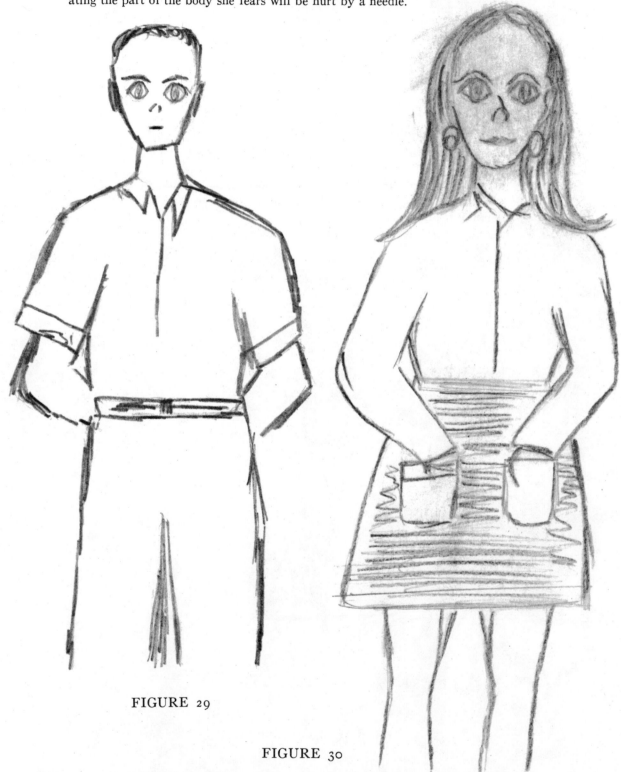

32

FIGURE 29

FIGURE 30

G.I.   *Age 14*   *Male*

The patient suffers from nasal allergies. His father and sister have colitis. Nothing remarkable was noted in his life history or appearance.

Drawings: These two figures are excellent examples of aggressive eroticized wish fantasies. The virility and physical strength of the male are over-exaggerated, almost caricatured in the beard stubble, fists and heavy hardware on the fashionable belt. The emphasis on the pectoral muscles and the presence of the ring add exhibitionistic touches. Underlying doubts about strong masculinity, to be expected in a 14-year-old boy, break through in the double lines and erasures seen on the trousers.

The female has a huge bosom, undoubtedly important in the boy's fantasy life. Her arms are strikingly short, hence ineffectual. The male is certainly the physically dominant one in this pair.

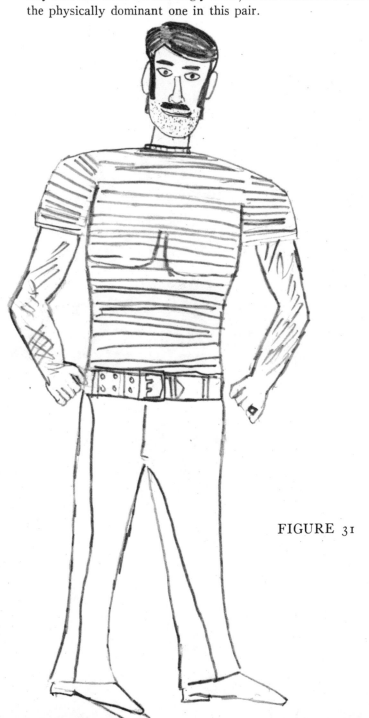

FIGURE 31

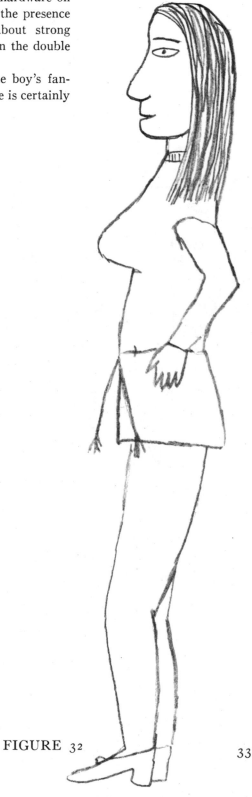

FIGURE 32

33

G.J.   *Age 17½*   *Male*

The patient suffers from spastic colitis. He is about to leave home for the first time to attend an out-of-town college. He is tense but pleasant, feels that he is "nervous" like his mother. He has been compliant, outwardly unaggressive all his life. He attributes his lack of social success with girls to his extreme thinness.

Drawings: They are far more atypical and immature than his history and interview would lead one to expect. He drew a girl first, differentiated from the male only by longer hair and the suggestion of body curves. Both have crossed eyes and large teeth, indicating anger and marked unconscious aggression. The concave mouth and buttons on the boy signify great dependence. Both have phallic noses and the outstretched arms of little children. The girl has fewer than five fingers, the boy has none.

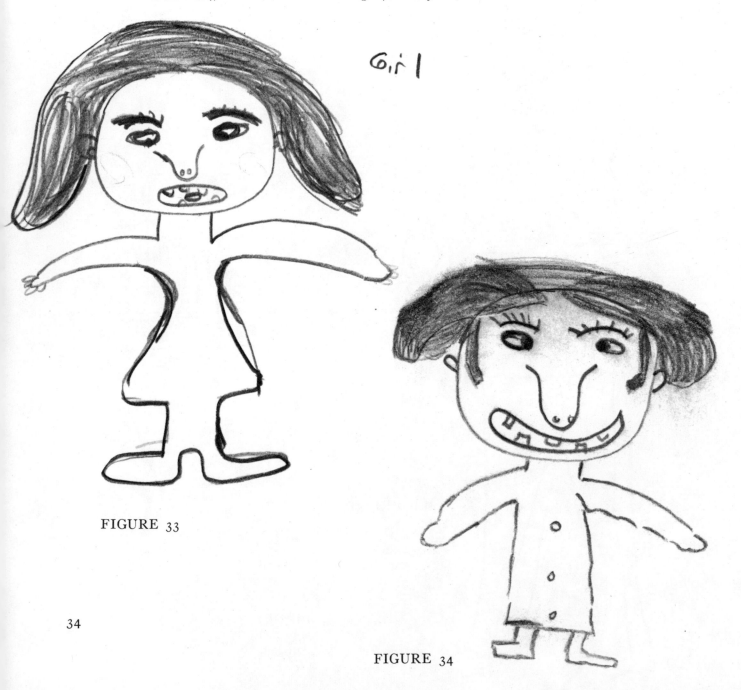

FIGURE 33

FIGURE 34

34

Two months later the patient remarked that he was feeling better and could improve on the previous drawings. He reversed the order, doing the male first. The essentially immature, oral aggressive, disproportionate character remains. The outlines are now more forceful, the boy's hair more masculine from an "establishment" point of view. The eyes are not crossed. The girl is younger, more pleasant, perhaps a shift from an angry mother image to a desired mate. The patient is right—there is some improvement, if one studies the details carefully. The original set of drawings was not available to him when he drew the second set.

The diagnosis of passive-aggressive personality disorder is strongly supported by the drawings.

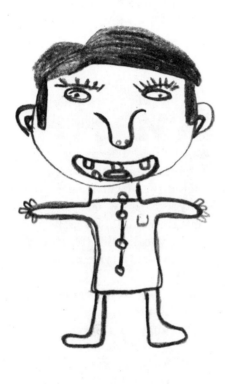

FIGURE 35

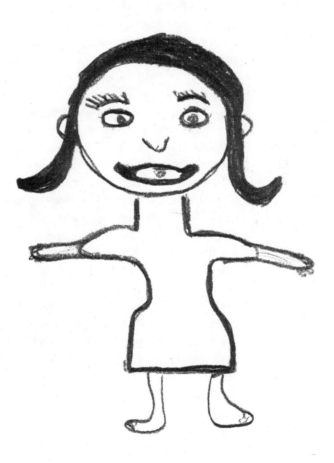

FIGURE 36

CHAPTER IV

Sexual Identity

Adolescence is, above all things, the time of life when each individual has to come to terms with the implications of his biological gender and the assumption of his sexual role. This does not imply that he has been in a neuter state all the years before. The psychosexual stages of his development have been unfolding since his birth, in a rhythmic or dysrhythmic pattern depending on the circumstances of his endowment and of his life. Through the processes of incorporation and identification with others he has integrated into his personality countless traits, gestures, movements, vocalizations and thought content which give him his particular individual style: masculine, feminine or ambiguous.

During the six to eight year span of adolescence, we see enormous development in the sex specificity of the human figure drawing, as demonstrated in Figures 50 and 51. This is due not only to a developmental growth in drawing dexterity discussed in the chapter on normalcy, but also to heightened awareness of sex-specific details. The drawings reflect the stage-specific as well as the highly individualized anxiety felt by many adolescents regarding their sexual identification. Wish fantasies, fear of sexual inadequacy, longing for the idealized body and masturbatory guilt are all projected. Defensive maneuvers against forbidden impulses appear again and again while seduction and aggressive hostility may be seen to coexist. Oedipal strivings, which are normally rekindled in early adolescence, are beautifully illustrated in Figures 39 and 40.

Much has been written about the significance of drawing one's own sex first, since the choice is left open to the patient. In well over 90% of our large sample, the adolescents do a human figure drawing of their own sex first. In younger children the incidence is much less. A study by Phelan among 6th grade boys (11-12 years old) did not show any difference in maladjustment in two matched groups. Adolescent girls, preoccupied with their sexual attractiveness, have a greater tendency than boys to draw an idealized figure of the opposite sex. Boys who draw females first are often expressing feelings about strong mother figures. Those who draw a more seductive type of female first are found to be more concerned with their own sexual identity and attractiveness.

Current youth culture attitudes towards a "unisex" appearance are amply illustrated in the choice of clothing (pants for girls) and the treatment of hair (long for boys), but are belied by the heavy emphasis on breasts in females. The possibility of a homosexual tendency is sometimes picked up in a human figure drawing. Here again, we would caution against using the human figure drawing as an exclusive diagnostic tool. It is, however, highly useful in helping us to explore the adolescent's feelings about sexuality in general and, in particular, to understand how he sees his own development in this most vital aspect of life.

B.A.   *Age 19*   *Male*

The patient came to the clinic complaining of a recent excessive loss of hair. Because of it, he has become anxious and withdrawn.

Drawings: The male figure shows emphasis on close-cropped hair and on the genital area, while detail is totally missing in the hands and feet. The figure has the appearance of a hanging puppet, reinforced by excessive attention to buttons which denote dependency. The shading and hesitation in drawing the left arm underscore the patient's anxiety.

The female figure is much larger, threatening, more human. The overpowering quality is neutralized by the absence of feet and the hidden hands. The nose is far more phallic than the clown-like button nose seen on the male. The hair and breasts are prominent. The heavily shaded clothing reveals the patient's anxiety about the opposite sex.

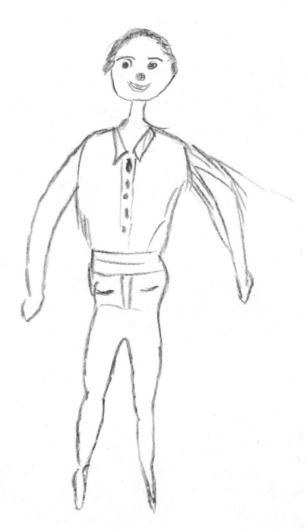

FIGURE 37

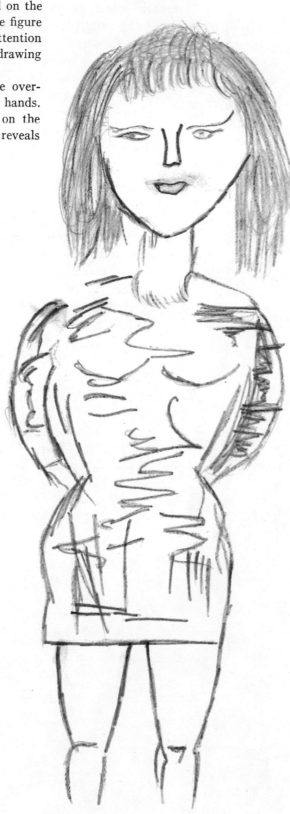

FIGURE 38

B.B.   Age 14   Female

This girl, a middle child, was brought to the clinic because of her demanding, willful, impulsive behavior. On one occasion she was suspended from school for drunkenness. Temper tantrums are severe and include physical assault. The patient stated that she "deserves being hit by mother" when she is disobedient. The dynamics of this masochistic remark become apparent in her drawings.

Drawings: The figures are well drawn. The female suggests seduction tempered by conflict, illustrated in the unusual crossed leg stance. The disproportionately large head of the girl shows immaturity and possibly a wish to have her head control her impulsivity. The hidden hands of both figures imply guilt and safeguards against sexual acting-out.

The male figure is older, bald, mustached. He appears to be unshaved and perhaps a little mean. The single wavy line dividing the trouser legs again demonstrates sexual anxiety. The tightly held together position of the legs in both figures is of obvious significance.

The drawings, looked at in the context of the girl's impulsive rage and expressed wish for physical punishment from her mother, point to an unresolved oedipal conflict. Her unconscious forbidden sexual wishes directed towards an older man (father) lead to guilt, displaced rage, impulsivity and anxiety.

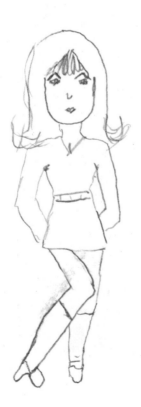

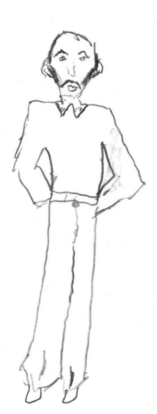

FIGURE 39   FIGURE 40

B.C. Age 13 Male

The patient came to the clinic for treatment of obesity. He denied having any other problems.

Drawings: The patient draws a skinny scarecrow type of male and pathetically labels it "male I think." He feels empty, weak, puppet-like. The unusually long neck implies that his mind is too far away from his body to adequately control his impulses, mainly in the area of overeating. He denies his obesity in the slim figure and straight-line closed mouth. He, in effect, castrates himself by drawing only three fingers and a minimal pelvis. The rigidly held arms and legs, close to the body, indicate marked ego restriction.

The female's body has such a faint outline as to be almost invisible. Her stereotyped face is darkly outlined, showing that his anxiety and avoidance have to do with her body. The female's arms reach out, possibly expressing a wish that she overcome his passivity. Her left foot resembles a paddle and her legs are separated, in contrast to the male's, indicating more elaborate sexual fantasies.

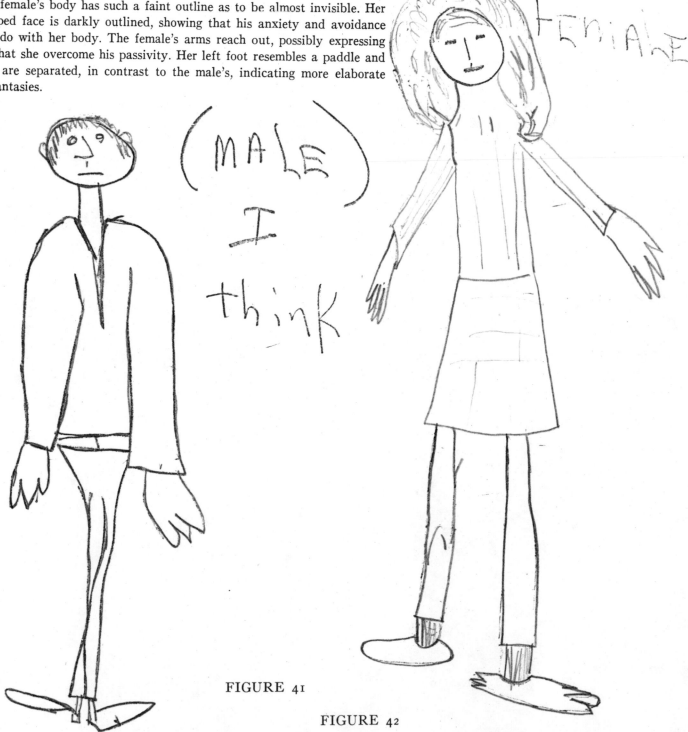

40

FIGURE 41

FIGURE 42

B.D.   *Age 19*   *Male*

The patient complains of seasonal allergies. No other significant data was elicited.

Drawings: The male figure is drawn lightly and indecisively. There are erasures and changes in the position of the right hand and foot. The left hand is but a stump and only three fingers remain on the altered right hand, implying feelings of guilt and castration anxiety. The female, in sharp contrast, is larger, drawn with heavy pressure on the pencil. Her clothing is heavily shaded, yet transparent and revealing. She is freer and more mobile than the male. The heavy emphasis on hair, enormous breasts, thighs and detailed knees are all projections of sexual impulses. The patient avoids clarity in drawing the female's hands, perhaps in this way neutralizing his evident anxiety that she is far stronger than he.

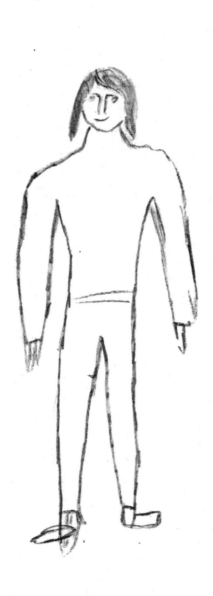

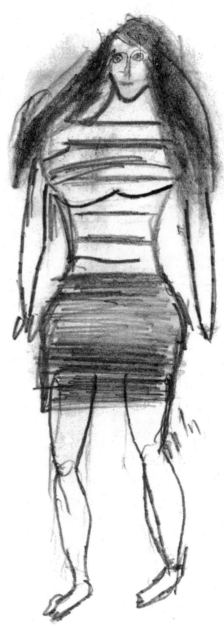

FIGURE 43

FIGURE 44

FIGURE 45

B.E.   Age 16   Male

The patient came for the treatment of acne, a condition he has had for several years. Although there has been some improvement, he cannot see it. He is in psychiatric treatment because of depression, irritability and severe conflicts with his father.

Drawing: Patient drew only the top half of a male (?) and refused to draw a person of the opposite sex. Fear of sexuality pervades his entire effort. The huge face covered with acne appears frightened. The glance is downward. The large nose is phallic. The sensual mouth is agape, ready to be fed or to scream. There is hardly any neck and the short arms extend outwards in an ineffectual, infantile manner. All the detail is concentrated on the face. The drawing clearly projects his inability to identify with a masculine figure, perhaps because of an unresolved oedipal conflict.

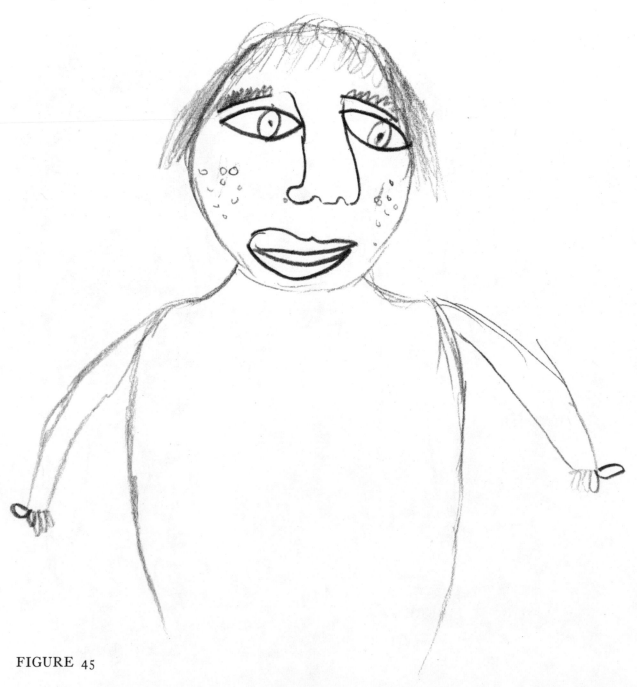

42

FIGURE 45

B.G.   *Age 15*   *Male*   *Follow-up 20 months later*

This patient came to the clinic for treatment of juvenile acne. Nothing unusual was uncovered in his life history.

Drawings: The normal struggle of a youngster striving for a strong masculine identity is beautifully demonstrated in these figures. At 15 he draws a tough looking man in profile. The right hand, executed with less skill than the rest of the drawing, appears to be making a negative gesture such as "nix" or "nothing doing," perhaps to the female. Notice that broken lines, characteristic of anxiety, are more prominent in the trouser area.

Turning to the female figure, we see that the boy had great difficulty in executing it. She is anonymous, buxom, disproportioned, missing many vital parts. On a second attempt, he again erases a great deal, totally omitting the head which is apparently not of much interest to him.

(*Continued on next two pages*)

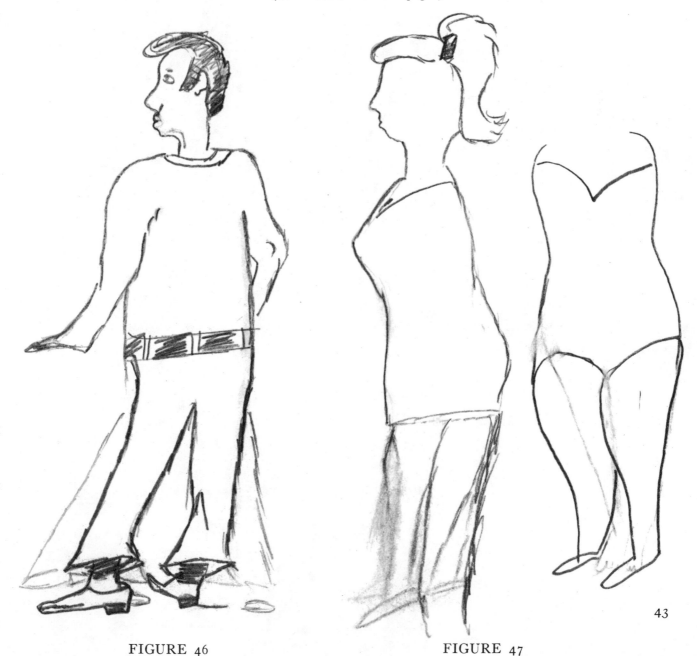

FIGURE 46   FIGURE 47

43

Twenty months later, now 16½ years old and more skillful, the youth has obviously defined his idealized body image. He has evolved into an enviable muscular lifeguard type, probably performing balancing stunts for the enticing lady in a bikini enjoying a delightful pool scene. The decorations on the male's bathing suit are appropriately placed for emphasis. Is the female holding Eve's apple? (*See next page.*)

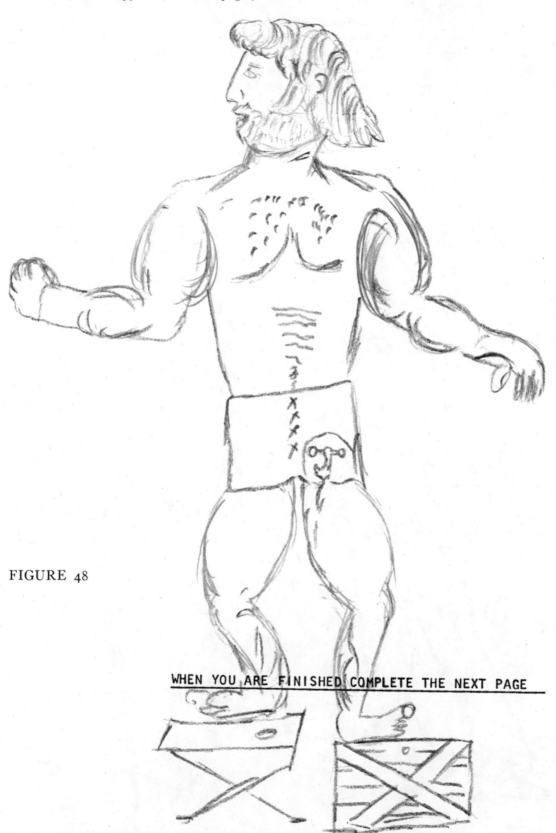

FIGURE 48

WHEN YOU ARE FINISHED COMPLETE THE NEXT PAGE

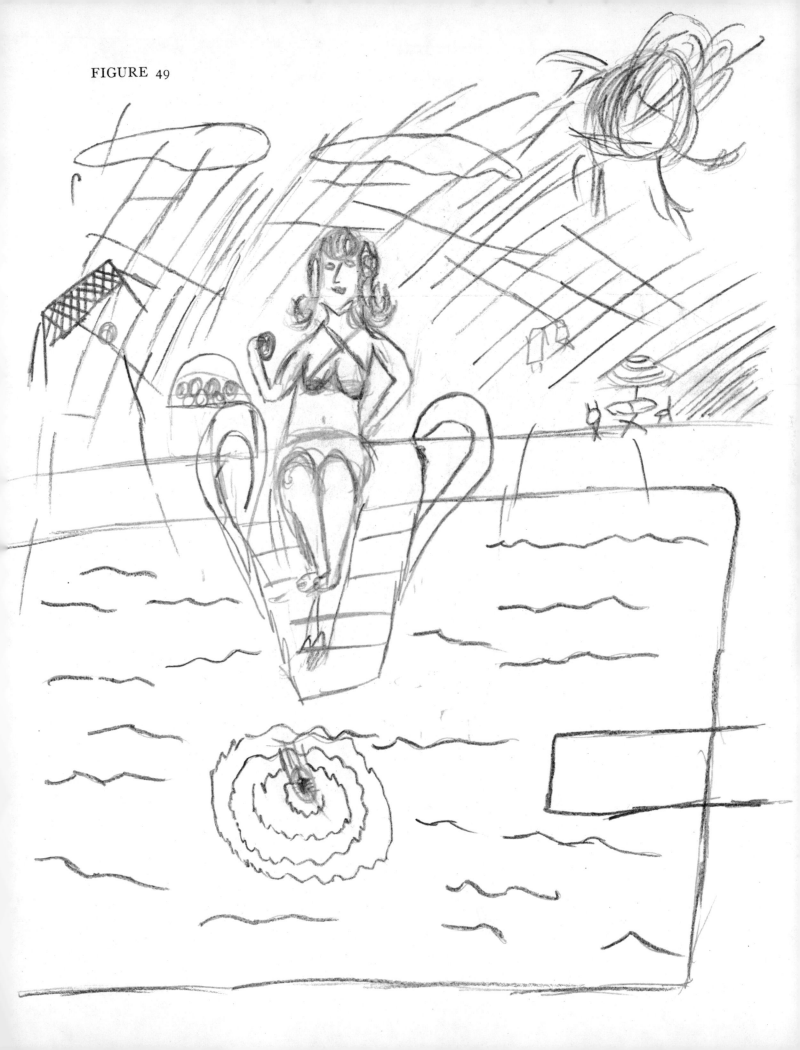

FIGURE 49

FIGURE 50

B.H.   Age 13   Male

This sample was collected from an eighth grade class of "normal" adolescents who were, like the patients, simply asked to draw a whole person. Nothing is known about the boy, except what the drawing tells us.

Drawing: We will limit ourselves to pointing out only the most significant features of this fantasy-rich production. The figure is bearded, virile, and tatooed with a girl and an anchor. There is activity emanating from every body orifice. The penis appears to have a huge padlock overlying it. The balloon he is blowing up is probably a condom. Feces pour out of the anus into a pot below an erect tail. Even the spigot in the sink is releasing fluid. Electrical attachments to the head give him extra exciting power. It is not difficult to conclude what is on this young adolescent's mind!

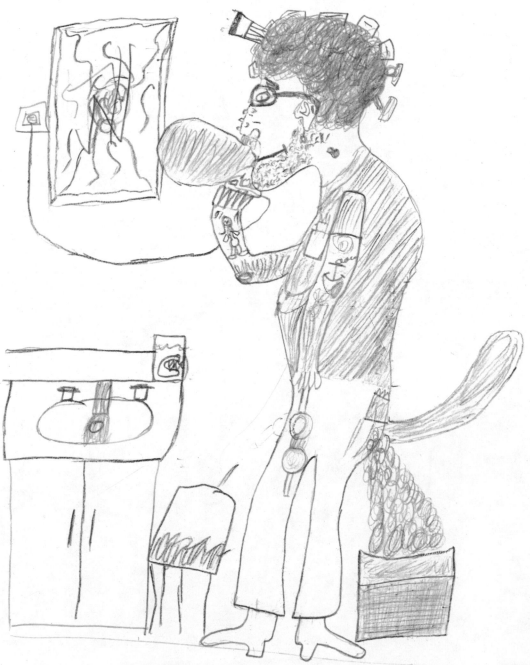

46

FIGURE 50

B.F.   Age 16   Male   Verbal I.Q. 141, Performance I.Q. 90

The patient came to the clinic for neurological evaluation, which was negative. His school work fluctuates from good to very poor. He is easily upset, has no friends, and is awkward in sports. He is generally well behaved. Psychological testing revealed an extraordinary degree of intratest scatter, depression, paranoid ideation and possible suicidal tendencies.

Drawings: Totally nude figures with explicit genitalia are rare, although less so than in younger children. In this disturbed, withdrawn adolescent, the content of some of his fantasy life, as well as his voyeuristic impulses, becomes evident in his human figure drawings. The nose of the male is a penis, that of the female a vagina. The ears are omitted, cutting off significant sensory contact with the outside world. The concrete representation of the elbows and knees is unusual, perhaps intended to humanize and mobilize these rigid figures. He is confused about the placement of female curves. The facial expressions are stupid, as he sees himself.

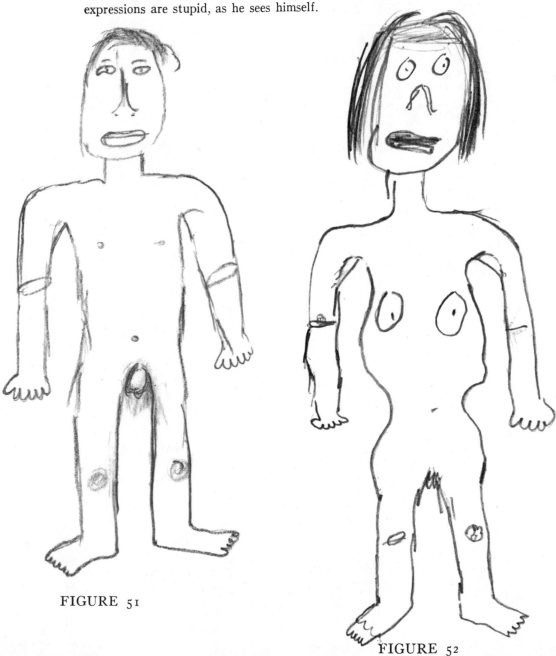

FIGURE 51

FIGURE 52

47

B.I.   *Age 17*   *Female*

The patient came to the clinic complaining of anemia and irregular menses. Her father, a hypochondriac, left the home two months ago. The patient feels confused.

Drawings: Gross immaturity is combined with sexual curiosity and preoccupation. The girl's dress transparently reveals tiny hanging breasts. Pubic hair (?) peeks out from under her dress. The asymmetrical arms emerging from the neck lack hands, reflecting the patient's feelings of being incapable. The nose is huge, the eyes lack pupils and the mouth has a bland fixed smile. The figure of the boy is similarly infantile and defective. His penis is blatantly exposed.

It is highly probable that this patient has deep psychopathology. Indeed, her menstrual irregularity may well be secondary to emotional problems. She sees herself as a small child despite her 17 years.

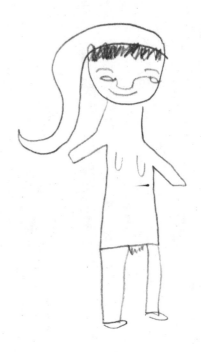

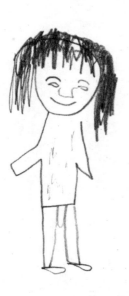

FIGURE 53   FIGURE 54

CHAPTER V

Physical Illness

Adolescence is both a physiological and psychological formative period. The normal "tasks of adolescence" are stress producing for all youngsters. The teen-ager who is undergoing the development of an adult body needs to adapt to his new self-image. The rapidity of growth and development which are occurring is only exceeded by those changes which occurred in the first year of life. A relatively homeostatic organism is suddenly disrupted by an outpouring of hormonal substances which effect dramatic changes in the adolescent. The altered endocrine state causes a marked increase in height and weight, and burgeoning of secondary sex characteristics with new body sensations. Accompanying these physiological events is a heightened awareness of peers and a need for acceptance by both the same and opposite sex, often conflicting with a desire to draw back to the comfort and security of childhood. It is in this charged state of emotional development that the onset of a physical illness upsetting normalcy tends to promote dependence at a time when independence is so vital. The real or imagined threat to the body image during adolescence can be more traumatic and difficult to cope with than at any other time of life.

It is our impression that the human figure drawings obtained from adolescents who are hospitalized for illness are reflective of the disturbed body image which they are experiencing. The drawings may aid in uncovering unsuspected conflict and anxieties, enlightening the physician or allied health worker treating the patient. A most striking aspect of this group of drawings is the projected feeling of being helpless and manipulated.

Human figure drawings are influenced by the large group of psychophysiological illnesses in a variety of ways. They may be helpful in confirming suspicions of a psychosomatic etiology for such common complaints as headaches and abdominal pain. Unconscious denial and difficulty in verbalization of feelings are common in these patients. The patient with a more significant organic illness may also be unaware of the conflicts he is experiencing, yet may project them through his human figure drawings. Attention is frequently concentrated on the afflicted part of the body.

Chronic illness in adolescence is especially tragic. It is emotionally unacceptable to patient, family, and staff. The death of an adolescent patient causes a subdued and grief-stricken atmosphere. Other patients may become withdrawn and negativistic and refuse medication. There is often no more challenging patient to deal with than the hospitalized adolescent. His needs are devouring, his hostility open, his demands insatiable, his protective denial of his serious illness tenuous. The following illustrations are examples of the human figure drawings of adolescent patients treated for various medical conditions.

D.A.   *Age 14*   *Male*

The patient was admitted to the hospital with swollen glands, pallor and fatigue. Diagnosis of acute lymphoblastic leukemia was made and the patient started on anti-leukemic medication. He had been ill for several weeks prior to admission.

Drawings: The patient draws typical armature figures indicating feelings of being non-human, manipulated by others. This type of drawing may be transient in nature, reflecting the concerns of the moment. The undifferentiated "female" figure is faceless. Drawings show depression, emptiness, suspicion, all of which are reality based in light of the patient's physical condition. The rigid armature may reflect an adaptive attempt to deal with overwhelming anxiety, by not allowing it to reach full consciousness.

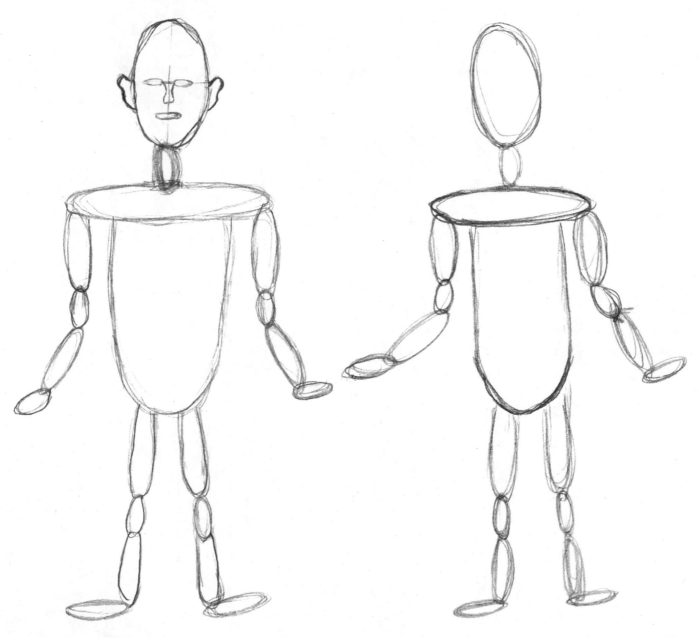

51

FIGURE 55   FIGURE 56

FIGURES 57, 58

D.B.   *Age 13*   *Female*

Patient is a Negro girl who has cystic fibrosis diagnosed at 7 months of age. She requires constant medication and supervision. Chronic illness severely restricts her life.

Drawings: The patient's body image is surprisingly intact and mature for a child who has been ill since birth. The girl leans on a heavy cane, as she does on medical therapy in real life. The constricted mouth is related to the dietary and respiratory restrictions of the disease. The pleated skirt, although fashionable, points to anxiety about the lower half of her body. Erasure of the cane and arm reveals her uncertainty. Obsessional trends are present in both drawings.

The male figure stands rigidly, perhaps because he is unavailable to the patient. Erasures in the trousers, in essence constricting the figure, point to sexual anxiety. The emphasized tie is phallic in implication. The abundant dark hair is culturally oriented, but also implies sexual excitement.

It should be noted that chronically ill patients, bedridden or sedentary, usually seek substitute gratification in a rich compensatory fantasy life.

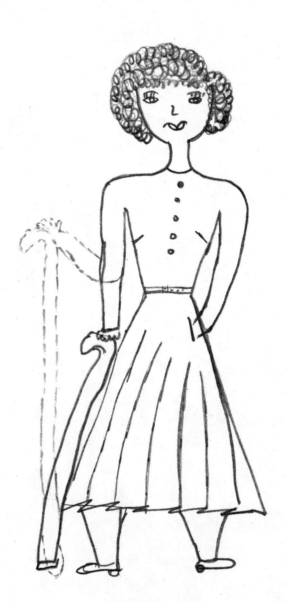

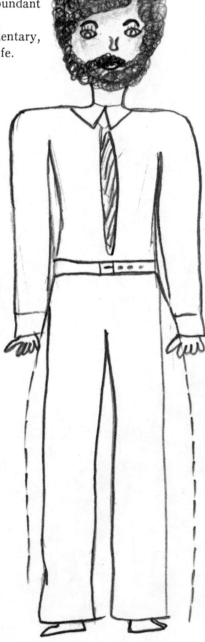

FIGURE 57   FIGURE 58

D.C.   *Age 17*   *Male*

The patient has had recurrent leg pains for many months. A benign bone tumor of the leg, osteoid osteoma, was diagnosed and the patient admitted for surgical removal of the involved area.

Drawings: The male is again noted to be of the armature type. The hand placed on the leg area of the knee is of obvious significance. The heavy shading reveals intense anxiety. The profile position shows a wish for avoidance. The face seems to be appealing for help and is slashed by several cross-hatched mutilating lines.

The female figure is aggressively in motion. She shows the sexual interest and anxiety characteristic of this age group. The unusual disposition of heavy hair surrounding the flirtatious face is indicative of sexual excitement.

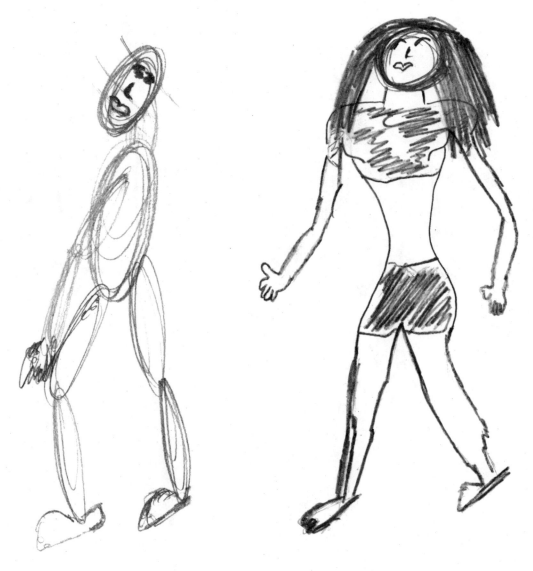

FIGURE 59   FIGURE 60

FIGURES 61, 62

D.D.   *Age 13*   *Male*

The patient has urinary tract symptoms: hesitancy, interruption of stream, and an episode of discolored urine. He is known to have minimal brain damage with mild intellectual impairment.

Drawings: These are clownlike. The outstretched fingers indicate aggression and possibly destructive impulses. Emphasis on the fly of the trousers is undoubtedly significant in light of the patient's symptoms. Obsessional detail of clothing is associated with concreteness of thinking. There is effort at impulse control indicated by the large number of buttons. The large feet indicate acting out or phallic preoccupation.

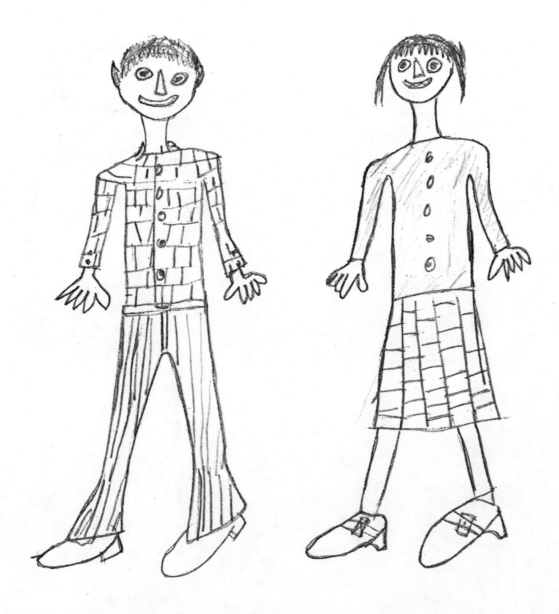

FIGURE 61   FIGURE 62

D.E.   *Age 13*   *Female*

Patient has Moebius syndrome which is characterized by ptosis of the eyelid associated with migraine attacks. She also suffers from incompletely corrected bilateral club feet and complains of leg pains.

Drawings: The patient draws heads that are disproportionately large, significant of her preoccupation with migraine headaches. The drawings are stiff, restricted and immature, the outstretched arms suggesting a baby asking to be picked up. Most important are the stick-like legs and small squared off feet, which undoubtedly relate to her symptoms. The slanting of the girl's figure is a sign of her insecurity. The transparent leg lines toward the center of the body reveal somatic preoccupation and poor integration. Dependency buttons are noted on the female figure. Inadequacy and helplessness are revealed by the presence of only three fingers.

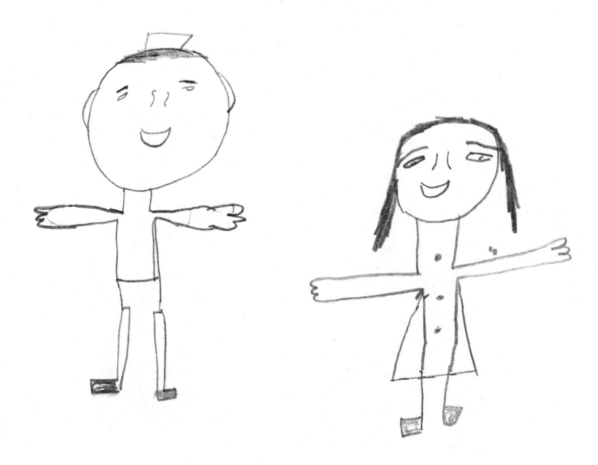

FIGURE 63   FIGURE 64

D.F.   *Age 15*   *Female*   *I.Q. 109*

Patient has been obese all her life. Many attempts at dietary control have been unsuccessful. The patient is moody and poorly organized. She is unable to sustain interest or effort in school.

Drawings: Lack of motivation is demonstrated in the first two stick-like drawings. When asked to put forth greater effort and encouraged to do so, the patient produces excellent mature drawings with faces in profile indicative of avoidance. The result is an idealized girl with a very good figure, much in contrast to her own body. One hand is hidden and there is pelvic shading. The drawing of the boy is effeminate. The broken lines indicate anxiety. The second set of drawings represents a wish fantasy, while the stick figures reveal how readily she regresses.

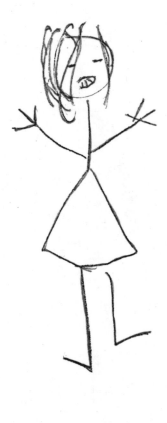

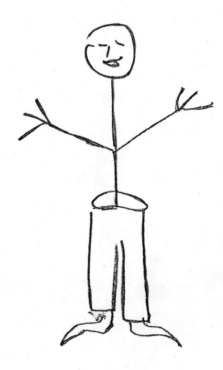

FIGURE 65   FIGURE 66

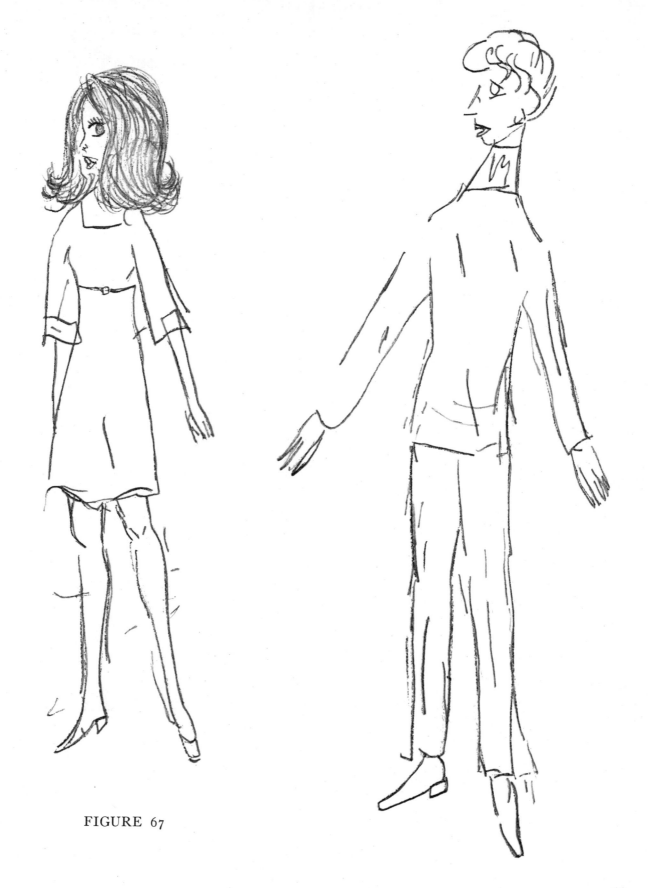

FIGURE 67

FIGURE 68

FIGURE 69

D.G.   *Age 13*   *Male*   *Average Intelligence*

Patient has been hospitalized for a duodenal ulcer. His mother has chronic mental illness, his father is a perfectionist who rarely communicates with the boy. Siblings and patient fight a great deal. He is disinterested in school, often doodles during class and has no friends. He is quite withdrawn and difficult to interview.

Drawing: Patient drew only one figure, although requested to do two. On being questioned about the sex of the figure, he replied, "I don't know—a boy." The figure is grossly immature, pseudo-retarded. Of greatest interest is the elimination of the lower half of the trunk, thus avoiding representation of the area of his somatic pain. The flaring nostrils, teeth, outstretched fingers and club-like legs all point to intense rage. The prominent ears are consonant with the possibility of auditory hallucinations, hinted at by the patient in an interview. The long neck is characteristic of obsessional ideation.

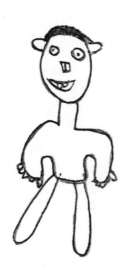

FIGURE 69

D.H.   *Age 20*   *Female*

Patient has severe cardiac disease which required the insertion of a permanent pacemaker. She has been hospitalized many times and is now an EKG technician.

Drawings: The patient draws a smoking male first, perhaps representing a wish to be a man or to have one. Both figures are drawn with the face in profile, indicating defensive avoidance. Of greatest interest is the necklace-like line on both male and female. It draws attention to the chest, obviously the area of greatest somatic preoccupation for this cardiac patient. The omission of hands and feet on both figures underscores her feelings of being "castrated," in a sense helpless because of her bad heart. The shaky outlines reveal anxiety. The omission of the pupil of the eye projects a wish not to see a painful reality. The emphasis on hair is both cultural and indicative of sexual excitement.

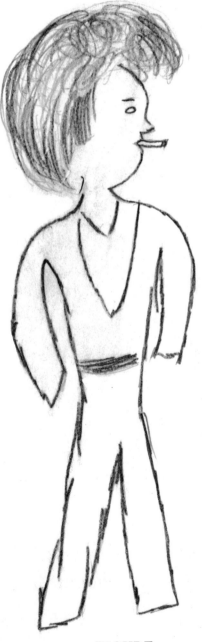

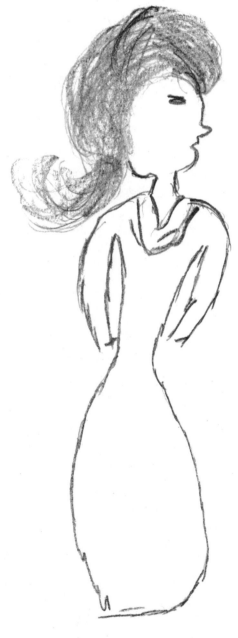

59

FIGURE 70   **FIGURE 71**

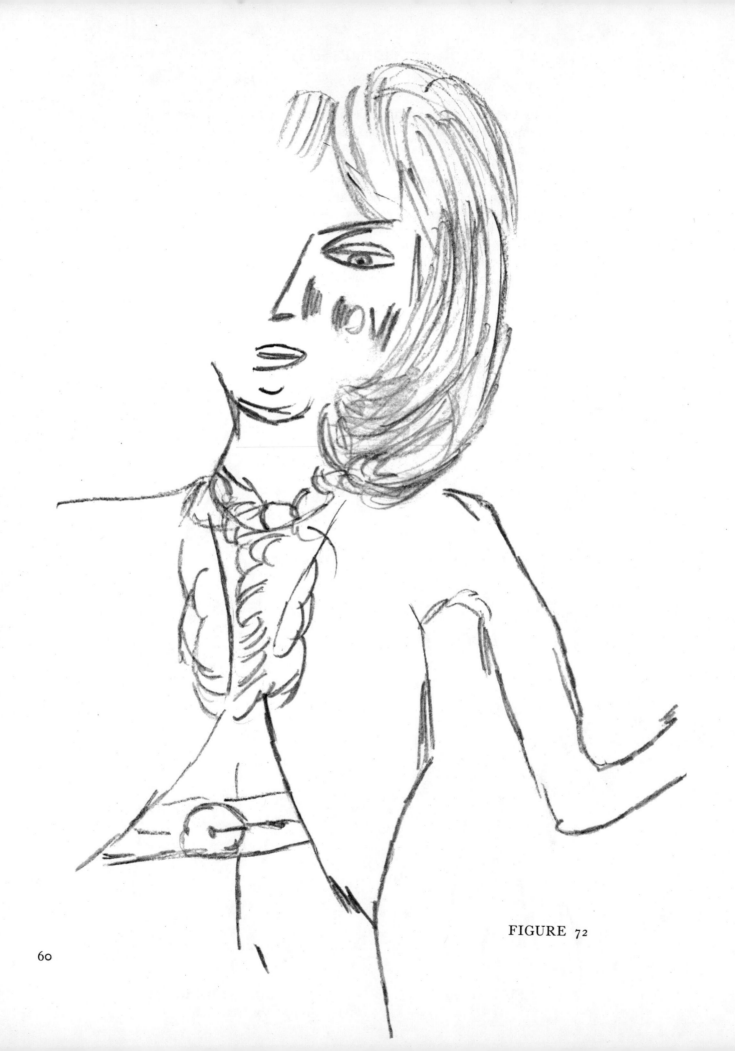

FIGURE 72

D.J.   *Age 18*   *Male*

The patient was admitted to the hospital for the surgical correction of prognathism (protruding lower jaw). He also suffers from a spastic colon. His parents and siblings are riddled with illness: diabetes, hypertension, coronary disease and mental illness.

Drawings: There is a marked difference in the techniques of the two drawings, and in their levels of maturation. The patient drew a female first, possibly his mother. The right side of her face and body are omitted, as well as the lower half of her body and left hand. This type of global omission demonstrates a state of extreme anxiety over body integrity, which one would expect in a family threatened by multiple major diseases. The shading of the left cheek is probably related to specific anxiety concerning the patient's impending mandibular surgery.

The male drawing is readily acceptable as a self-portrait. The distorted face has a huge jaw concealing the neck. Is he wearing a surgical gown and cap? The right hand appears to be waving good-bye. The drawing is of much poorer quality than the first, a reflection of how the patient feels about himself. The shading and slashing lines are further evidence of anxiety about body mutilation.

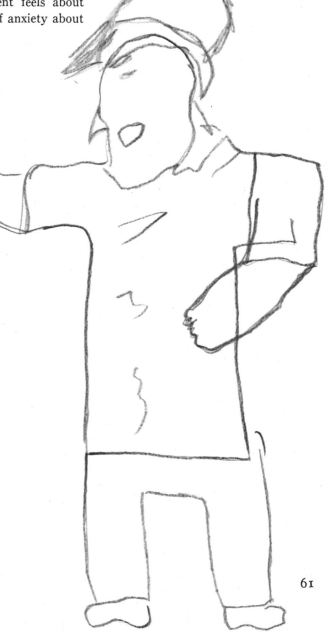

FIGURE 73

61

FIGURES 74, 75

D.K.   *Age 13*   *Male*   *I.Q. 89*

The patient has multiple physical handicaps, including dwarfism and subtotal blindness. He is diagnosed as having Morquio's Disease, spondyloepiphyseal dysplasia congenita, and is only 3 feet tall.

Drawings: They are compensatory in size. There is significant absence of the eye in the male and an absence of the pupils in the female. The figures are Frankenstein-like monsters, either a projected wish to have such power or the way he perceives himself or others in the world around him. The female's big teeth make her particularly threatening. The absence of detail is correlated with his immaturity, low average intelligence and lack of visual acuity. He seems to feel empty. The broken lines, especially in the outline of the male, reveal intense anxiety.

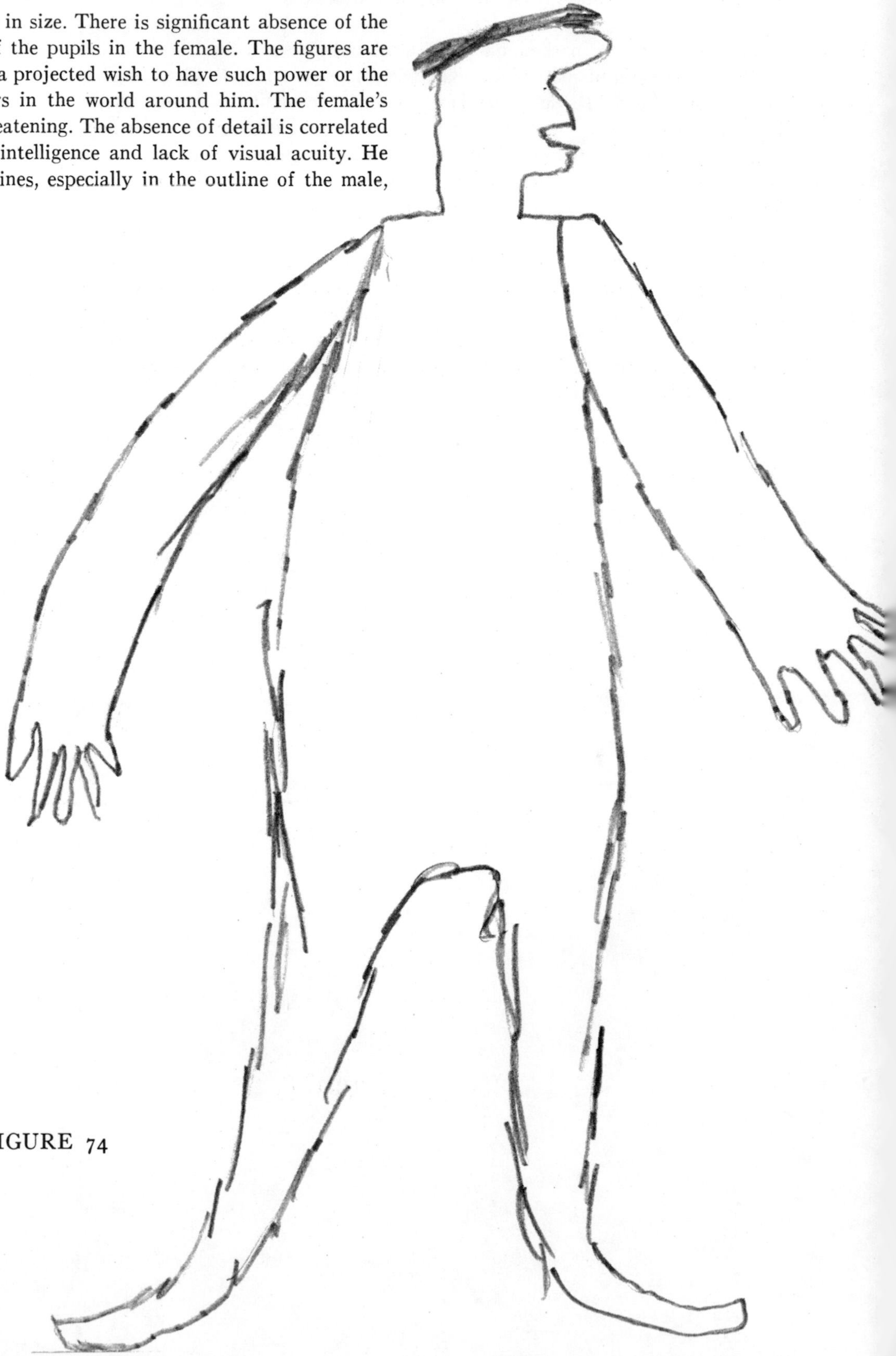

FIGURE 74

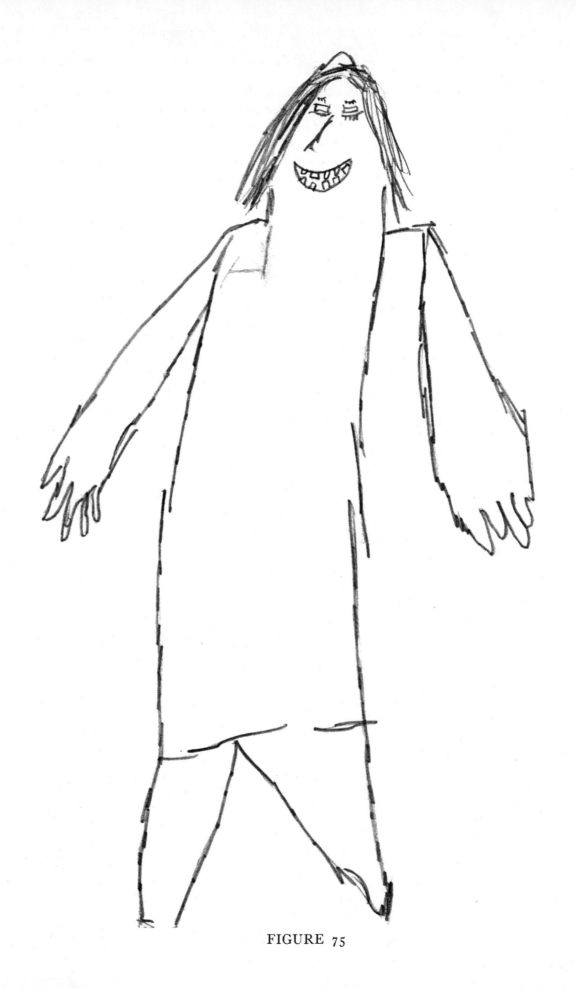

FIGURE 75

FIGURE 76

D.I.   *Age 15*   *Male*   *Superior Intelligence*

Patient was born with arthrogryposis, a condition characterized by multiple joint deformities. He has had many operations and was admitted for further corrective surgery, which he refused. Psychiatric consultation revealed that he feared anesthesia and was disappointed with the results of last year's operation. He is extremely anxious about his future in every respect.

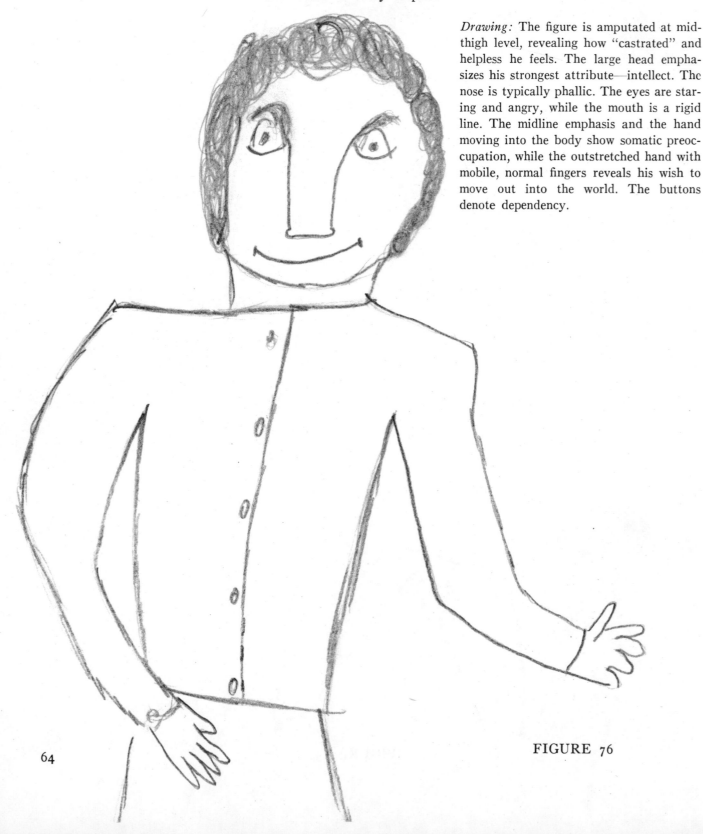

Drawing: The figure is amputated at mid-thigh level, revealing how "castrated" and helpless he feels. The large head emphasizes his strongest attribute—intellect. The nose is typically phallic. The eyes are staring and angry, while the mouth is a rigid line. The midline emphasis and the hand moving into the body show somatic preoccupation, while the outstretched hand with mobile, normal fingers reveals his wish to move out into the world. The buttons denote dependency.

FIGURE 76

D.L.   Age 18   Male

The patient has a history of ulcerative colitis of 5 years duration. He has undergone ileostomy and colectomy and now has a perineal sinus.

Drawings: They are extremely dependent and immature. The lower half of the body is omitted, thus eliminating the troublesome gastro-intestinal tract. The figures are poorly integrated. Some degree of oral fixation can be inferred from the miniature breasts of the female and the large, open mouths. The attenuated figures and short arms, without hands in the case of the boy, reveal his feeling of inability to perform. The disproportionately large heads point to obsessional ideation and perhaps the feeling that only his head has worth. Upward genital displacement is seen in the way he differentiates between the noses of the male and female. Only the male is suspended above a potentially supportive base line.

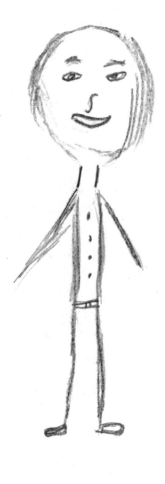

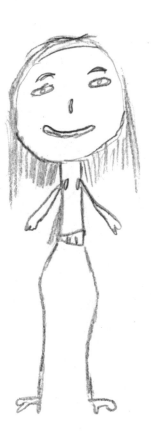

FIGURE 77   FIGURE 78   65

FIGURES 79, 80

D.M.   *Age 19*   *Male*

The patient was admitted to the hospital because of a large testicular swelling. He was operated on and found to have a testicular tumor.

Drawings: These were obtained one week after surgery. It is obvious that he is concerned with the genital area, protecting it with hands in both the male and female drawings. The crossed legs of the male heighten the inaccessibility of his swollen, vulnerable testes. The girl's thumb suggests a phallus. The heavy shading of the clothing and the ground line, although appropriate, are signs of anxiety. The male figure has a worried facial expression.

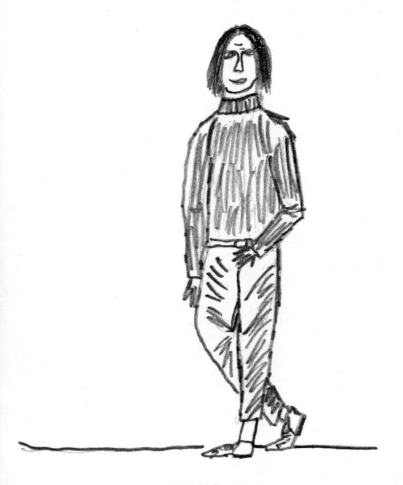

FIGURE 79

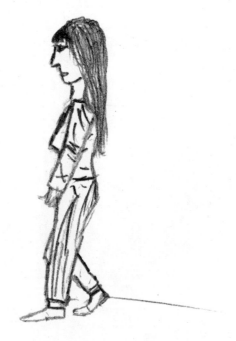

FIGURE 80

66

FIGURE 81

D.N.   *Age 14*   *Male*

The patient suffers from gynecomastia. He is embarrassed by his large breasts and tried to hide them during the examination.

Drawing: Contrary to his behavior, the drawing clearly emphasizes his problem breasts. The clenched fists reveal his anger. The lower half of the figure is masculine and virile.

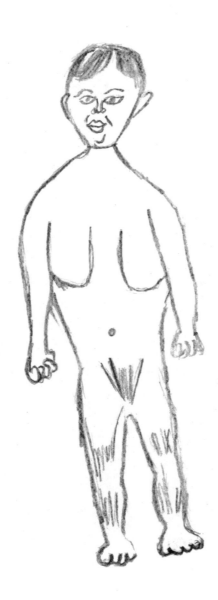

FIGURE 81

D.O.   *Age 12*   *Female*

The patient has a congenital heart condition, about which she verbalizes no concern.

Drawings: The globular body of the female is manifestly heart-shaped. From the shoulders upward the drawing is of much better quality, although immature. The similar small floating figure of the male shows intense concentration on the cardiac region. Neither one can see, lacking pupils.

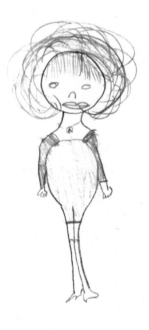

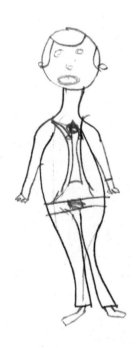

FIGURE 82   FIGURE 83

CHAPTER VI

Organicity

The diagnosis of organicity, a term broadly used to indicate all types of neurological deficit, draws strong support from certain qualities in the drawing of the human figure. Indeed, there are many experienced diagnosticians of differing disciplines who are willing to venture this diagnosis presumptively on the basis of such drawings alone. It is not, of course, possible to refine such a diagnosis by so simple a test. A drawing may, however, alert the observer to investigate further, especially when the patient's complaints are vague, denied or absent.

In recent years there has been a growing trend to use the term "organicity" to imply the presence of "minimal brain dysfunction." This is a syndrome, not uncommon in children, characterized by hyperactivity, poor fine motor coordination, short attention span, uneven maturation and other subtle deficits, especially in cognition. We deplore the use of these terms as interchangeable. In point of fact, minimal brain dysfunction is simply one type of organicity, requiring fairly subtle tests and clinical acumen to diagnose. The human figure drawing is, in our opinion, a most useful diagnostic tool in the evaluation of this problem. The exact nature of minimal brain dysfunction is still poorly understood. Current studies point towards a genetic, physiological basis. Hypoxia leading to venous thrombi and prenatal viral lesions have also been incriminated. It is clear that the trouble is not anatomically localized. Most children burdened with this disorder improve functionally over the years, probably through learned compensatory cerebral mechanisms. The I.Q. may or may not be impaired and children with high intelligence may be so afflicted.

Emotional problems are invariably present in varying degree, because of the child's feelings of inadequacy in simple coping skills and in his sense of difference. Adverse environmental reactions and lack of success may intensify the emotional component to such a degree that it predominates. The syndrome is far more common in males, hence the preponderance of drawings done by boys in our series.

No single type of drawing is characteristic of the organically impaired adolescent. The regressed, retarded organic patient will often produce a drawing difficult to distinguish from those done by childhood schizophrenics. A feature common to most organic patients is their feeling of disorientation in space, often displayed in their drawings. We consider the following findings as most characteristic of organicity, especially when they appear in clusters. No single one is in itself pathognomonic and no single one is present in all cases.

1. Gross immaturity of drawing.
2. Poor integration of parts.
3. Emptiness of facial expression.
4. Lack of details.
5. Omission of parts, especially the neck.
6. Transparent or absent clothing.
7. Flattened heads.
8. Displacement of the extremities.
9. Petal-like or scribbled fingers and toes.

What is striking about this group of drawings is that they all demonstrate some degree of maturational arrest. None are characteristically adolescent. There is virtually no growth change in patients age 12 to 18. Sexual differentiation is rudimentary. These patients see themselves as sticks, segmented balloons, puppets or squared-off robots. Even when these patients improve clinically through the administration of drugs, psychotherapy and improved management, their drawings retain a basic "organic" character.

A.A.   *Age 12*   *Male*   *I.Q. 85*

A.A. is an obese boy, the youngest of five children, suffering from a severe speech defect and reading disability. His fine coordination and handwriting are poor due to a manual tremor, intention type. He has elderly parents who infantilize him. The patient denies having any problems despite his difficulties in school, home and the peer world.

Electro-encephalogram is negative. There is no explicit etiology of his condition other than his mother's age, about 46, at the time of his conception.

Drawings: These are infantile, 6 to 7 year level. The large head represents denial of his problem and perhaps the wish for a better brain. Absent neck, squared body, downward displacement of arms and spindle fingers are typical of organic brain damage.

The female figure shows asymmetry of the lower extremities and absent upper extremities. Perhaps this expresses the patient's wish to rid himself of his mother's smothering attention.

Facial expressions of the drawings, bland and perpetually smiling, actually resemble the patient's mimetic style and are a clear projection of his defensive denial.

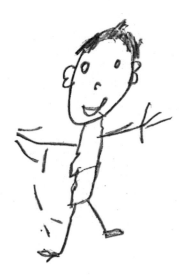

FIGURE 84

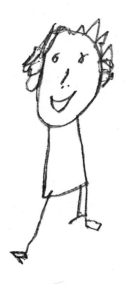

FIGURE 85

A.C.   *Age 12½*   *Male*   *I.Q. 92*

A.C. was referred to the clinic because of chronically poor school performance, enuresis, oppositional behavior at home and extreme sibling jealousy. He has a mild speech defect. His voice and appearance are flat and colorless, his movements are slow. The patient has crossed dominance. Electro-encephalogram is mildly abnormal.

Mother stained during pregnancy and took tranquilizers.

Drawings: Highly regressed, empty, transparent. The figures appear to float in mid-air. Figure 86 shows aggressive, outstretched, club-like hands. The eyes are empty, undifferentiated from the nose except for proper placement. Figure 87 shows preoccupation with breasts, revealing his voyeuristic impulses towards his older sister. The female lacks fingers.

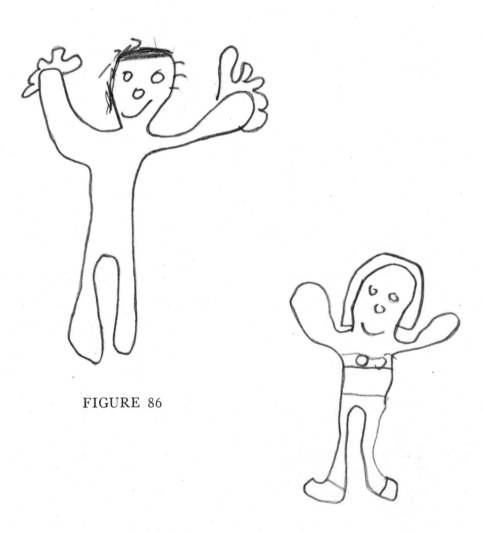

FIGURE 86

FIGURE 87

A second set of drawings done 4 months later shows a shift in defenses. The male face is drawn in profile, implying defensive avoidance of feeling. The arms no longer reach out, the hands have totally disappeared. Psychological testing correlated with the second set of drawings reveals the patient's attempt to control aggressive impulses through the establishment of compulsive rituals. Elimination of the hands holds sadistic and masturbatory impulses in check. The female has lost her distinguishing sexual characteristics, no longer presenting a seductive threat. The attempt to erase the second female figure shows his anxiety concerning her body and his wish to "undo" her. The two later drawings are done with a firmer line, corresponding to the feeling of a stronger base depicted in the more adequate feet on which the figures stand. Thus, the patient seems to feel more secure by developing defenses that keep his aggressive and sexual impulses in better control.

These drawings are an excellent example of organicity compromised by secondary emotional reactions and burgeoning sexual feelings.

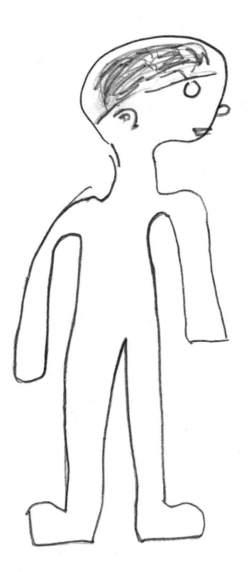

FIGURE 88

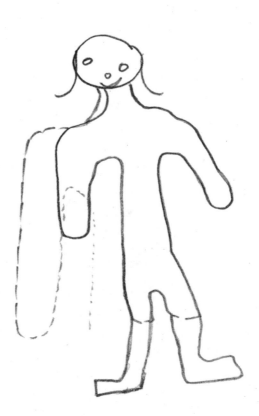

73

FIGURE 89

FIGURES 90, 91, 92, 93

A.D.   *Age 13*   *Male*

The patient was referred by his school because of inability to concentrate and remember, a speech impediment and reading retardation. His fine motor coordination is poor. He is unable to copy a square or a triangle. His gross motor coordination is good, enabling him to participate fairly well in sports. As a result, he gets along well with his peers, unlike so many children suffering from chronic brain syndrome.

Drawings: Immature puppet-like figures resemble scarecrows. The absent neck and outstretched arms are typical of the brain-damaged child who has a sense of poor inner controls. The pronounced midline emphasis and the presence of large buttons on the undifferentiated torsos indicate his need for dependency. The nose is absent in the first two figures, indicating feelings of castration. The fingers are like petals, the toes are spindles, both typical of organicity.

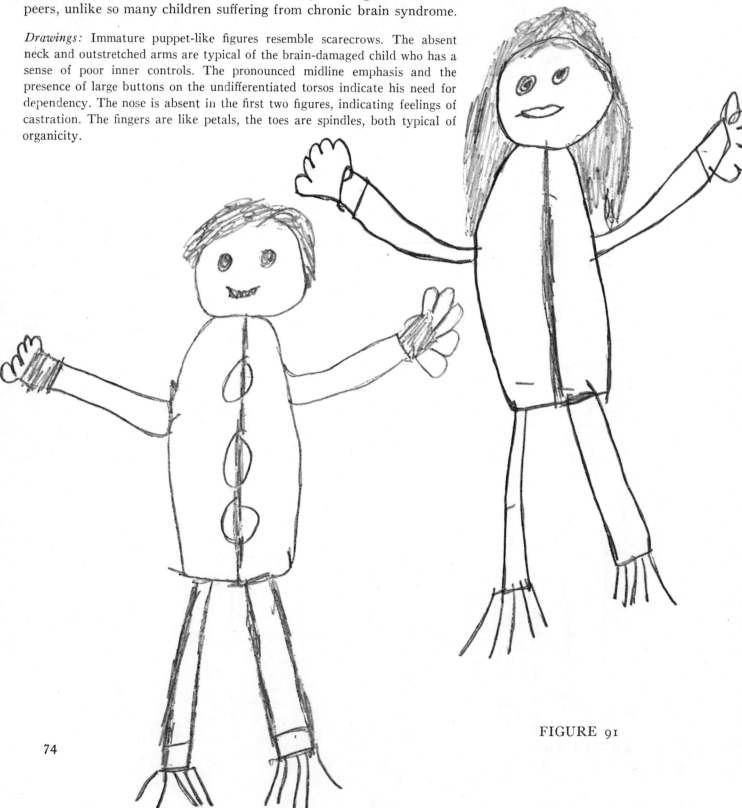

FIGURE 91

74

FIGURE 90

In the second set of drawings done two months later, the general character remains the same. However, the nose is now present, while the eyes are more vacant. The legs have become sticks with knobbed terminals, unfit to support the weight of the body. Although the patient was unable or chose not to copy a triangle on direct request, the second set of drawings reveals a compulsion to draw triangles, even when inappropriate, in the perseverative manner of the organically brain damaged.

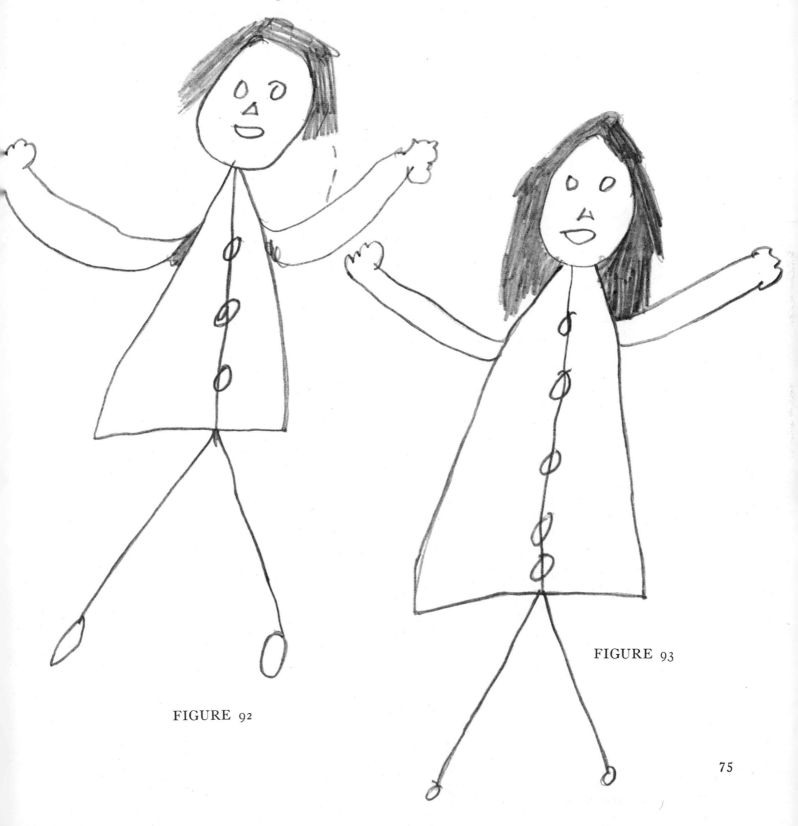

FIGURE 92

FIGURE 93

75

A.B.   Age 18   Male   I.Q. 70

Patient has diminished attention span, poor coordination and a speech defect. He is constantly in his mother's company, displays effeminate behavior, passivity and compliance.

Drawings: At first he drew stick figures, slashing the faces with poor control. He was easily persuaded to try harder. He then produced improved immature drawings, having more substance but still poorly differentiated. The female figure is weaker and smaller, indicating a wish for greater masculine strength. The absent neck is typically organic, immature. The ball-like hands and feet in the second set of drawings reflect his feelings of clumsiness and inability to do things.

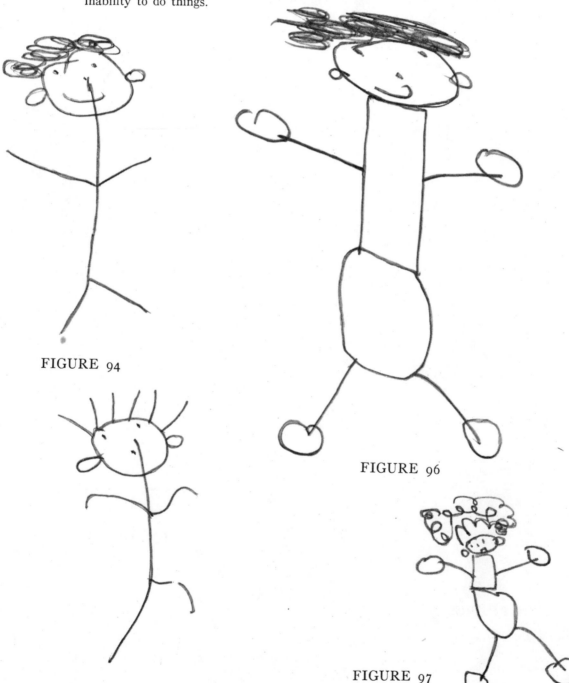

FIGURE 94

FIGURE 96

FIGURE 95

FIGURE 97

FIGURE 98

A.E.   Age 15   Female   I.Q. 50

Patient is a cretin, born of a hypothyroid mother who died at childbirth of rheumatic heart disease. Although treated with thyroid extract at an early age, physical and mental development have been markedly retarded. She is nerve deaf but has learned to lip read on a simple level. Despite these severe handicaps, the patient tries hard to learn, performs simple tasks and is generally well behaved and pleasant. She lives in an adoptive home with sympathetic parents.

Drawing: The patient's perseverative attempts to draw the human figure are at a relatively high level in respect to her diminished general ability. The lines are shaky, the details are poor, the arms are wing-like and displaced. Nevertheless she keeps trying, reflecting the goal tenacity she displays in real life. She does not attempt a figure of the opposite sex. The prominent presence of buttons reveals her dependency needs. It is of interest to note that the third figure gets smaller, reflecting her own diminutive size. Although the first two figures may show a wish to be of normal size, the discrepancy is more likely to be organically determined.

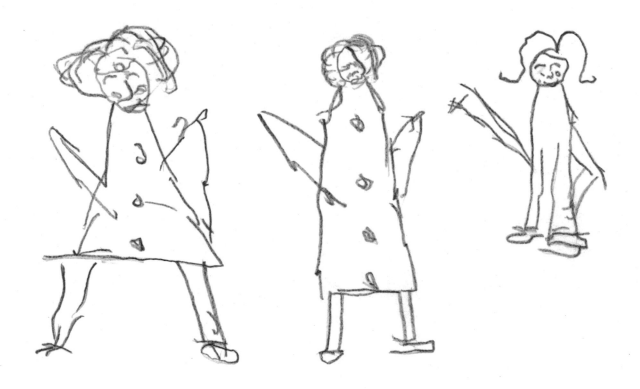

FIGURE 98

A.F. *Age 19* *Male* *Verbal I.Q. 80*

Performance I.Q. 63 *Full Scale I.Q. 71*

This patient was referred by the N. Y. State Department of Vocational Rehabilitation for evaluation of his suitability to learn a trade. He was found capable of doing more complex tasks while unable to do some simple ones.

He was born with clubfeet, asymmetrical ears, and partial paralysis of the lower lip. He has lived a very sheltered life, without friends, and has harbored many fears. He was recently graduated from a high school special class. The patient dresses very stylishly, apparently in an effort to compensate for his awkward, ungainly appearance.

Psychological testing, which he was reluctant to undertake, revealed considerable intra-test scatter attributed to both organic and emotional factors. The test demonstrated the patient's defensive exclusion of environmental detail from consciousness, in order to spare himself anxiety. The conclusion is that this young man, born with minimal brain dysfunction, could function at a much higher level if not for the severe secondary neurotic overlay.

Drawings: This 19-year-old youth draws two virtually identical stick figures, eliminating confrontation with awareness of the opposite sex. The primitive body has no genitality. Ears and feet are specifically excluded, since the patient's deformities of these parts are too painful to see. Indeed, the eyes do not see. The marked concavity of the large perpetually smiling mouth denotes oral dependency and denial. Aggressive impulses can be inferred from the club-like hands.

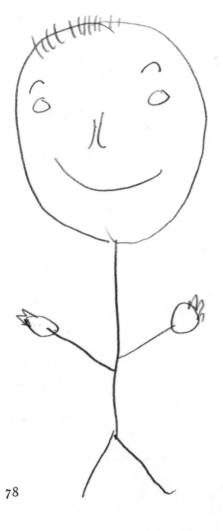
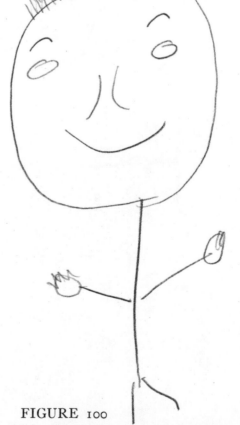

78

FIGURE 99 FIGURE 100

A.G.   *Age 16*   *Male*   *Average I.Q.*

Patient complains of a short memory, episodic feelings of being dazed, and recurrent severe headaches. He is considered to be lazy at home, difficult in school and has no friends. On occasion he has had fist fights and does not remember what provoked him.

Electro-encephalogram is abnormal, suggestive of a seizure disorder. Diagnosis: epilepsy, psychomotor type.

Drawings: Although organic, they differ markedly from the previous samples. Both male and female have a "zombie" quality. The eyes of the male have a paranoid sidewise glance. The bodies appear to be unclothed, except for the brassiere on the female, but there is no body detail. The light wavy outlines suggest uncertainty and awkward manipulation of the pencil. The arms are far from the body, clumsy and difficult to control. The hands are mere stumps. The female pelvis has bizarre bumps. Her feet are in profile pointing in the same lateral direction, while the body faces us in a rigid anterior position.

These drawings have a more mature quality than the previous ones illustrating organic damage. This patient has a specific problem: epilepsy. He does not show the maturational lag of the minimal brain dysfunction cases. Hence his drawings, although "organic" and defective, are adolescent in character.

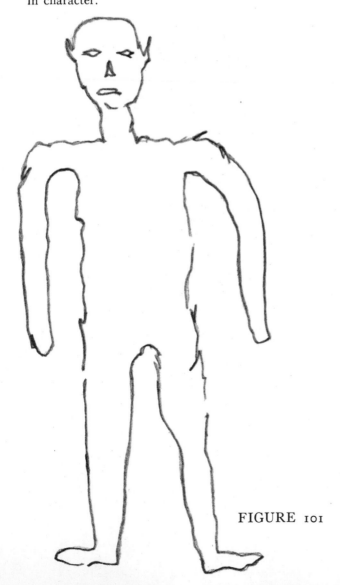

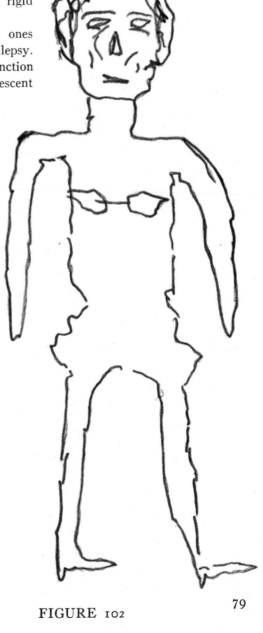

FIGURE 101   FIGURE 102

A.H.   *Age 14*   *Female*   *Average I.Q.*

This patient has had grand mal epilepsy for the past two years, controlled by medication. She is hypochondriacal. Parents were separated a year ago and patient has found it difficult to adjust to the absence of her father and to a new neighborhood. She clings to her mother.

Drawings: Patient chooses to draw a male first, probably because of longing for the absent father. The figures display her marked immaturity and feelings of helplessness. Without hands or feet, what can she do by herself? The female head is disproportionately large, an infantile characteristic. The female torso is too large for the pelvis and the stumps which substitute for legs. The shading denotes anxiety. The bland smile is a denial of her true feelings.

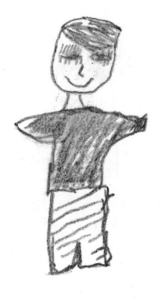 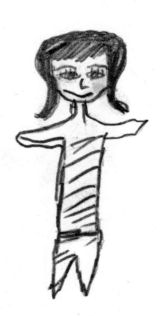

FIGURE 103   FIGURE 104

CHAPTER VII

Neurosis

In searching for signs of neurosis in the human figure drawings of our adolescent patients, we select primarily those characteristics which indicate the presence of anxiety, depression, obsession and guilt. Not infrequently, the patient projects onto his drawing some evidence of the mechanisms of defense which he unconsciously employs to protect his ego from the assaults of the id and superego, such as repression, avoidance, denial and reversals. In the chapter on psychosis we present material demonstrating the regressive perceptual distortions of the body image and the bizarre quality caused by breaks in reality testing. In this chapter the drawings demonstrate that, despite the intensity of the emotions experienced, the ego structure of these adolescents is sufficiently resilient to deal with conflict without resorting to significant regression. This difference between the neurotic and psychotic state of being is as fundamental in clinical understanding and prognostication as is the difference between the benign and malignant state of a tumor.

Machover has pointed out that interrelated patterns of drawing traits may reflect the dynamics of symptom organization in a particular diagnostic category and that drawings tend to overlap in the same manner as symptoms do in varying clinical syndromes. Hence, we remain constantly aware, in our selection of sample drawings, that our choice is based on a preponderance of suggestive traits such as shading, broken lines, erasures, asymmetry, slanting and other evidence of the possible existence of an underlying conflict. When these traits are picked up in the drawing of an adolescent with vague or seemingly unrelated complaints, it is a fascinating challenge for the clinician to explore the patient's history and emotional state in search of corroborative evidence of the existence of underlying neurotic conflicts and trends.

E.A.   *Age 14*   *Male*

The patient was referred by his school because of his erratic academic performance and frequent misbehavior. Since his parents' -divorce, he has been fighting with his siblings and his mother.

Drawings: Both figures are skillfully drawn "portraits" of the current youth culture. The young man looks depressed. Hidden hands imply guilt feelings. Broken lines of such intensity indicate anxiety. The voluptuous female is faceless, suggesting hostility or fear of a heterosexual relationship, in conflict with strong sexual attraction. Both figures are exceptionally mature for a 14-year-old. Circumstances surrounding parental divorce often stimulate sexual fantasies in the children.

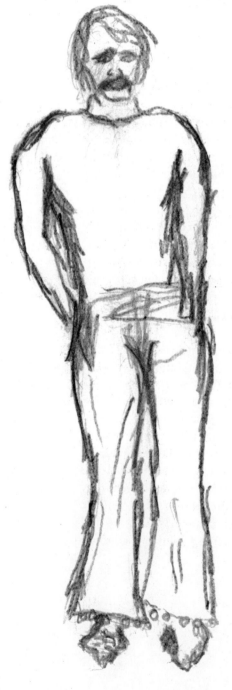

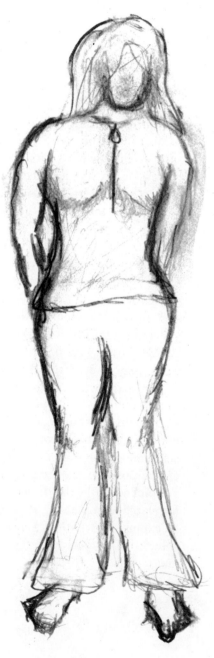

82

FIGURE 105

FIGURE 106

E.B.   *Age 19½*   *Female*

The patient came to the clinic deeply concerned about acne, excessive hair on her face and menstrual irregularity. She is socially withdrawn and uncomplaining. Her father died when she was 10 and she assumed the role of mother to her younger siblings, while her mother went to work and fell into the role of father.

Drawings: The patient sees herself as a sad, unapproachable duenna. Instead of facial hirsutism, genetic in origin, she draws a heavily shaded dark mantilla covering all but the smallest profile view of her face. The closely striped angular dress which reaches to the floor, even covering her toes, makes her impregnable.

The attractive male figure is seen in a frontal view. But he too is wearing a cape covering much of his body. The heavy shading in the opening of the cape testifies to the patient's anxiety concerning the opposite sex.

Drawings, life history and personality all tell the same story. Depression and anxiety are manifest.

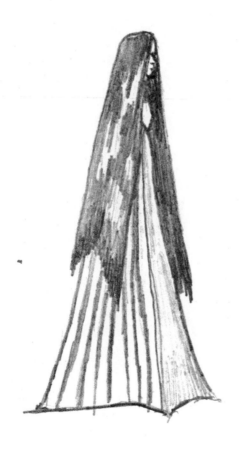

FIGURE 107

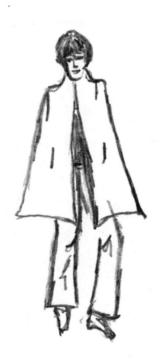

FIGURE 108

E.C.   *Age 17*   *Female*   *I.Q. 140*

The patient came to the clinic on the insistence of her parents who find her difficult to live with because she "chooses" to isolate herself and rarely communicates with them. Despite her very superior intelligence, she does very mediocre school work and has no goals. When, after some time, it became possible to establish some rapport with the patient, she expressed feelings of contempt for her parents, despair about herself, distrust of others and episodes of depersonalization.

Drawings: The skillfully sketched adult bodies are headless. This is a most significant finding since figure drawings, except in the most disorganized individuals, start on the top. Two interpretations may be made: feelings of anomie and a wish to eliminate the source of painful thoughts. The hands and arms are poorly executed in contrast to the skill exhibited elsewhere. The lightness of touch and incompleteness reveal her self-concept of ineffectualness. The strong male torso, genitally indefinite, is on his knees and appears to be imploring help from some divine or stronger source. It is a moving figure, reflecting some rich fantasy, perhaps a wish to dominate a man. Conflict and anxiety are apparent in the exaggerated broken-line technique and shading.

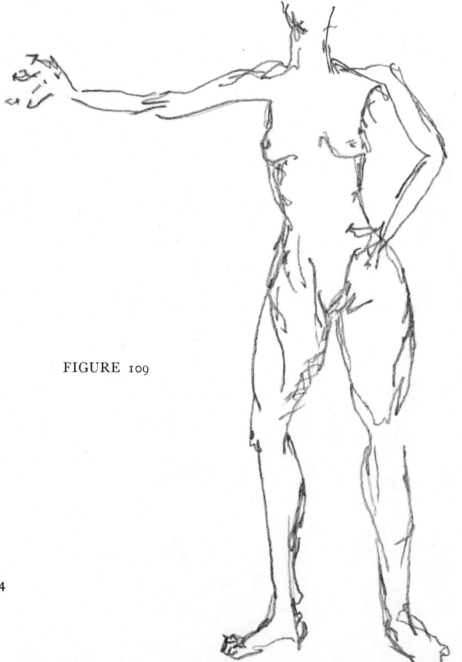

FIGURE 109

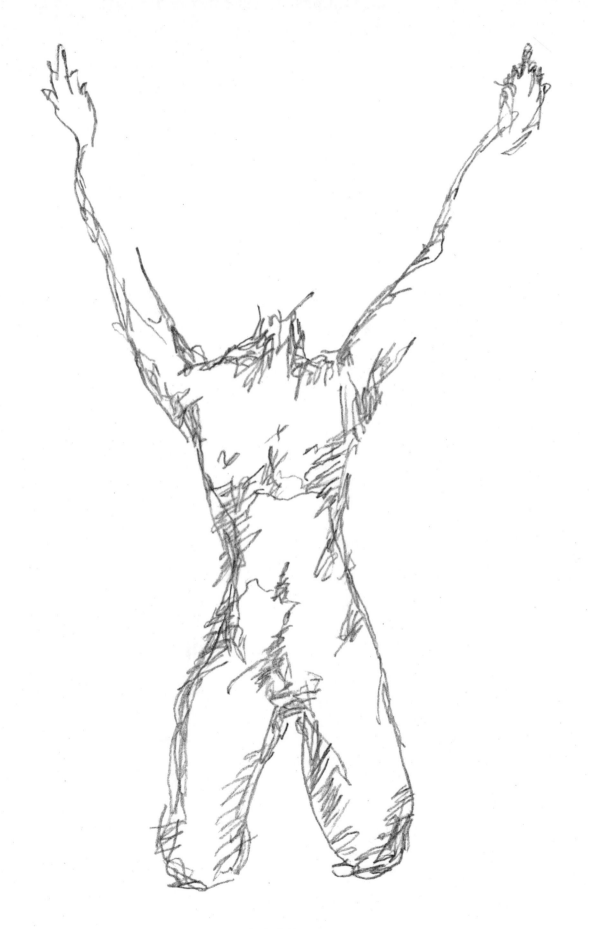

85

FIGURE 110

E.D.   *Age 17*   *Male*   *I.Q. 126*

The patient came to the clinic concerned about his uncontrollable temper. It takes very little provocation to make him assaultive. After an outburst, he feels guilty and ashamed. He is nervous much of the time. He fears his father "without reason." Sometimes he thinks he is getting paranoid.

Drawings: The shaky lines in drawing the male attest to his anxiety. The eyes lack pupils, making him "blind." This is, in a sense, how he feels when he flies into a blind rage. The right arm is rigidly immobilized at his side. The left is moving out, as though beyond his control. Interestingly, he is left-handed. The absence of feet has him immobilized—he cannot act out his impulses. This omission also implies feelings of being castrated, significant in a young man struggling with latent homosexuality. These interpretations were further supported by Rorschach findings.

The drawing of the female is more integrated. She too lacks feet. Machover points out that knee emphasis, as seen here, is common in homosexuality.

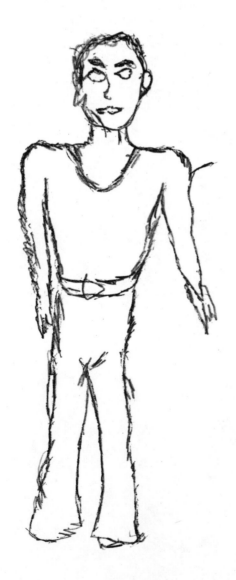
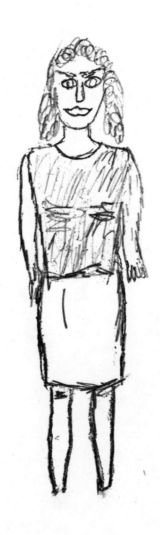

86

FIGURE 111   FIGURE 112

E.E.   *Age 15*   *Female*

The patient came to the clinic with exaggerated concern about a mild facial acne and irregular menses.

Drawings: Here again we see the adolescent project his overriding anxiety about his appearance. This girl eradicates her acne by becoming totally face-less. The boy is seen in profile, a sign of avoidance. The line quality is jagged, much less sure than in the case of the female figure. He lacks eyes to see the faceless girl and keeps his hand safely hidden in his pocket.

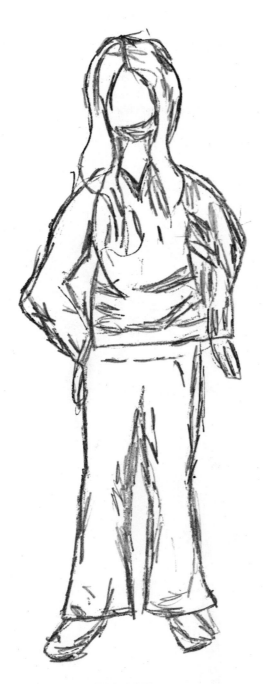

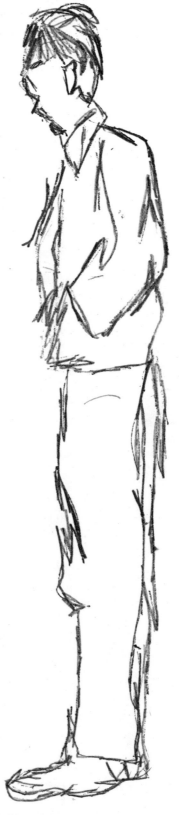

FIGURE 113   FIGURE 114

E.F.   *Age 13*   *Male*

This patient came to the clinic because of an enormous weight gain since his father's death a year earlier. Two foster sisters who had lived with the family for 11 years, and of whom he was very fond, left the home when the boy's father died. In school he has been clowning and joking and at home his mother reports that "he tends to be aggravating and exasperating."

Drawings: The figures are clown-like silly puppets, arms outstretched in limp curves as though waiting to be manipulated. The unusually heavy, inappropriate total shading indicates the patient's intense body anxiety. It is likely that his father's death has given him this powerless, depressed feeling. The thin-lined smile is an unconscious denial of such painful feelings. When over-eating is used as a defense against depression, as in this boy, it is invariably denied in the human figure drawings of our adolescent material. There are many immature omissions in this case: pupils, ears, nose, hands, all underscoring his impotent self-image. The figure of the girl shows more anxiety in the form of erasures and superimposed gashed lines. The music note type of legs seen on the girl shows more anxiety in the form of erasures and superimposed gashed lines. They are an unusual finding in a non-stick figure, adding to its sub-human quality.

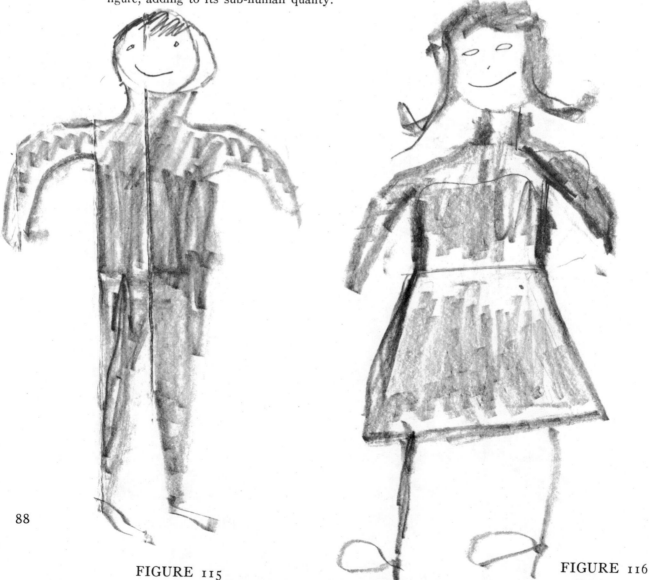

FIGURE 115   **FIGURE 116**

E.G.   *Age 14*   *Male*

The patient came to the clinic for evaluation of his short stature. He plays mainly with younger children. His relationship with his father is a poor one. He has been the recipient of frequent beatings.

Drawings: He drew a girl first, unusual in boys of this age group. Her stance is a very aggressive one. The arms, placed akimbo, terminate in huge outstretched hands. Knuckles, nails and joint markings are prominent. Omitting the feet neutralizes some of her aggressive potential. Shading, especially of the lower half of her body, and the light broken lines attest to his anxiety about girls, who obviously frighten him.

The male figure is drawn with a very dark line, in sharp contrast to the rendering of the female. It is obviously his father, on whom he wreaks vengeance by totally eliminating the lower half of the body, two fingers of the right hand and the whole of the left one. The face looks mean and cannot really see, lacking pupils.

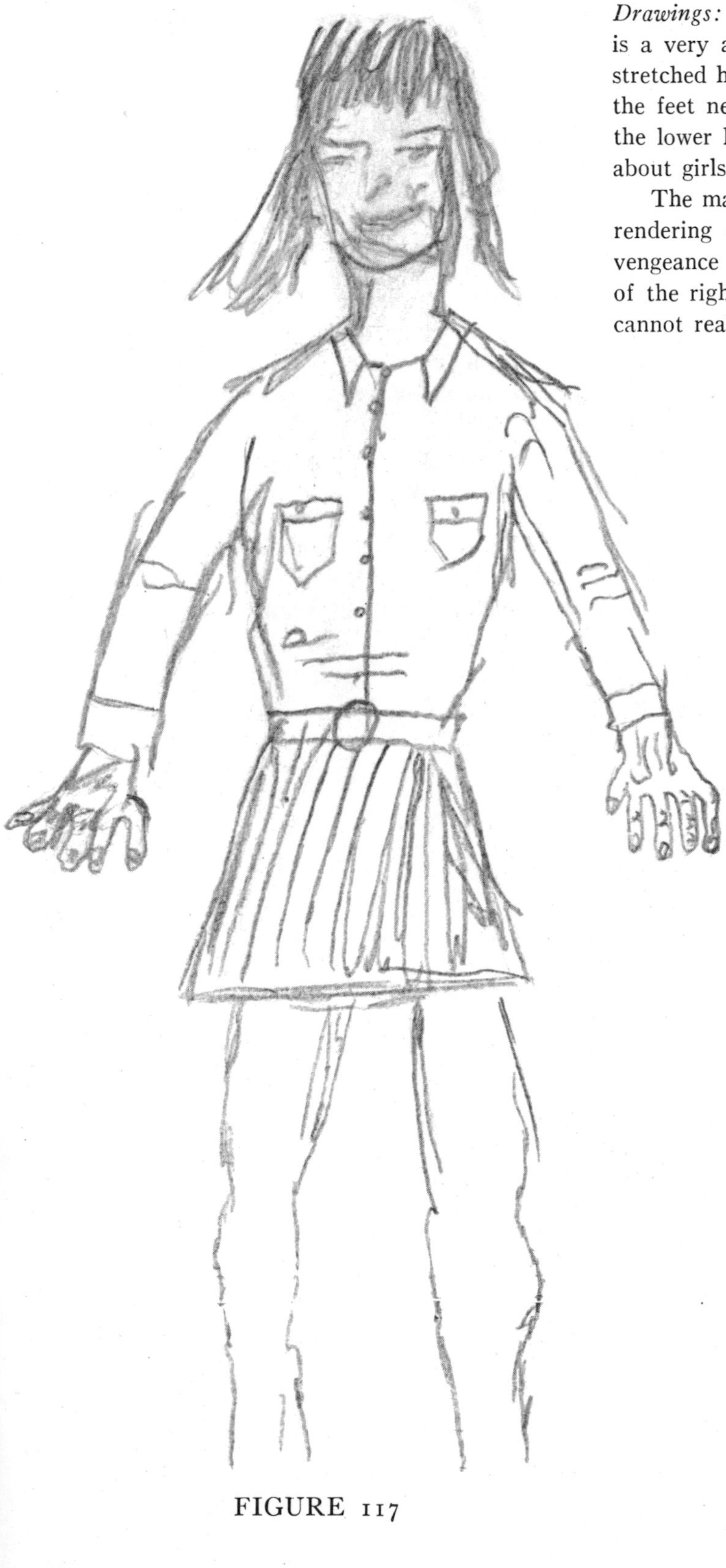

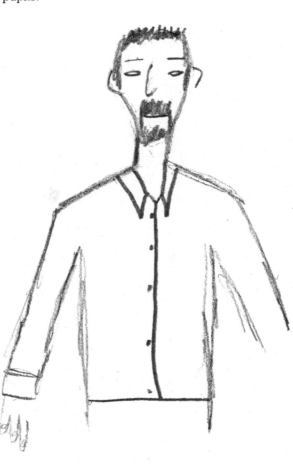

FIGURE 118

FIGURE 117

89

E.H.   *Age 12*   *Female*

The patient recently developed recurrent episodes of difficulty in breathing (hyperventilation syndrome) and feelings of gastric fullness. She is afraid to eat and stopped attending school a few weeks ago. The prospect of a physical examination throws her into a panic state. Her mother suffers from thyrotoxicosis and has had bouts of anorexia nervosa. The patient shares a room with her mother, while the father sleeps in a separate bedroom.

Drawings: The girl is seductive in an immature manner. The emphasis on hair indicates a state of excitement. The lips are full. The transparent dress reveals the breasts. Although this is currently fashionable, it also puts emphasis on the area of her body about which she is most concerned. The random scribbled shading is not uncommon in the hysterical personality. The left hand appears to beckon, while the right thumb points inward to the pelvis. The low-slung belt and buckle call further attention to this area. Conflict concerning sexual wishes is shown in the crossed legs.

The male figure resembles Manson, the California commune murder leader who at the time was very much in the news. He has a somewhat cruel look, in contrast to the "luv" and peace messages decorating his fringed bluejeans. The patient's sexual preoccupation is quite evident in the "69" drawn in the fly area and the "luv girls" at the bottom of the trousers. The right hand behind his back has to do with guilt or a sense of mystery.

From the clinical history and drawings we see that this 12-year-old girl's sexual fantasies are more than she can handle without recourse to hysterical conversion symptoms.

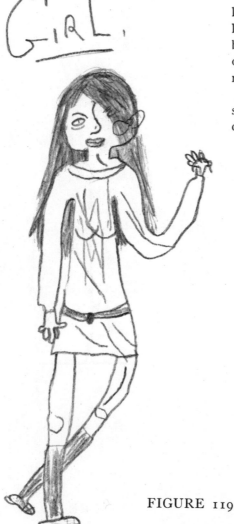

FIGURE 119

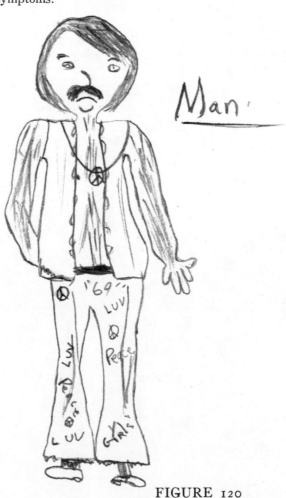

FIGURE 120

FIGURE 121

E.I.   *Age 15*   *Female*

The patient complains of headaches that last for hours. She lives in a foster home where she is very unhappy. She attacks her 2-year-old foster brother and resents her sister who is promiscuous. In a previous foster home, the father sexually molested the patient.

Drawing: Extreme anxiety concerning body integrity is demonstrated in the transparent female figure in which internal organs are depicted. In view of this anxiety, it is reasonable to interpret the presence of headaches as a neurotic conversion symptom. The absence of hair desexualizes the figure. Ears are omitted, partially cutting her off from her resented environment. The arms and legs are asymmetrical, the hands are hidden behind the back, rendering them less assaultive. The figure rests on a much needed base. Emphasis on the knees is said to indicate homosexual impulses. This would not be unexpected in a girl who had suffered a sexual attack at an early age.

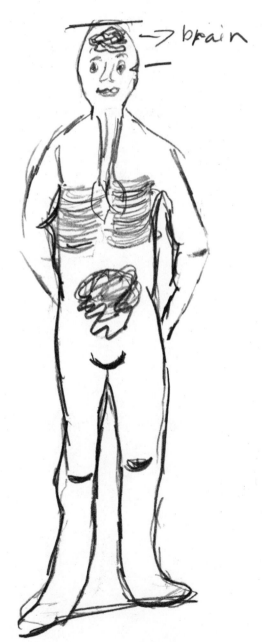

FIGURE 121

E.J. *Age 17* *Female* *Above Average Intelligence*

The patient came to the clinic for the treatment of juvenile acne suffered since she was fourteen. She is also allergic. Her school work is outstanding and her ambition is to be a psychologist. She is troubled by serious difficulties with her father. She is the only child of elderly parents of Sicilian background. The father forbids her to date and is suspicious of strangers. He doted on her as a little girl and is deeply angered by her attraction to "hippy friends," vegetarian food fads, etc. The parents will not even consider her wish to go to an out-of-town college. She feels guilty about her rebellion. The thought of marriage "sickens" her.

Drawings: The figures are poorly drawn for a 17-year old of superior intellect. The sun always "rose and set" on her in the eyes of her parents. We see it shining above the girl, but canceled out in obvious conflict above the boy. The girl is shown in profile, a sign of defensive avoidance. The large head corresponds to her intellectual ambitions. The facial expression is angry. Ears are missing, perhaps expressing a wish not to hear what her parents have to say. The arms are short and the hands are rudimentary, indicating her fear that she will not be able to do the things she would like to do. The heavy shading and broken lines reveal her high level of anxiety. The male figure has similar characteristics, but a smaller head and better hands. His mouth and torso are slashed, as though she would like to eradicate him.

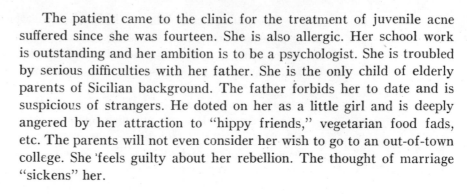

WHEN YOU ARE FINISHED COMPLETE THE NEXT PAGE

FIGURE 122

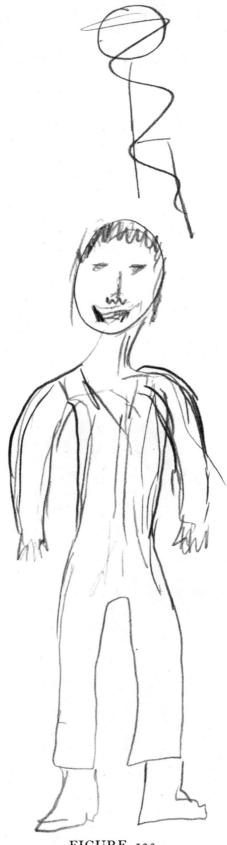

FIGURE 123

E.K.   *Age 14*   *Male*

The patient complains of irritability, listlessness, abdominal pains and headaches. He had refused to attend school for the previous two weeks. The parents are divorced. The mother complained that the boy is constantly quarreling with her and his sister. When a routine blood test was to be taken, the patient ran out of the clinic in a panic.

Drawings: The heavy shading on the male figure, despite its appropriateness in indicating clothing, implies considerable anxiety. The Afro hair style and mustache done by a white boy, although culturally overdetermined, reveals a state of sexual excitement (emphasis on "wild" hair). The convergent pupils or "cockeyed" look indicate that he feels confused, does not know in which direction to look. The arms are akimbo, puppet-like, implying that he feels controlled by outside forces. The emphasis on buttons, buckles and stripes suggests obsessional ideation and somatization.

The female drawing is not human at all. It is a heavily shaded Halloween type figure which he spontaneously labels "the wicked witch," revealing his hostility towards his mother and sister. The witch's nose is clearly phallic. It is likely that he sees his mother as domineering, cold and potentially harmful in a magical way, and that he blames her for the loss of his father. Witch figures are common in younger children, not in normal adolescents.

These drawings are highly consonant with the patient's current neurotic behavior.

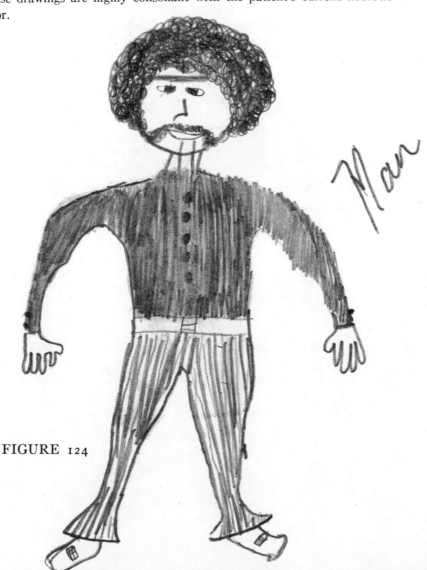

FIGURE 124

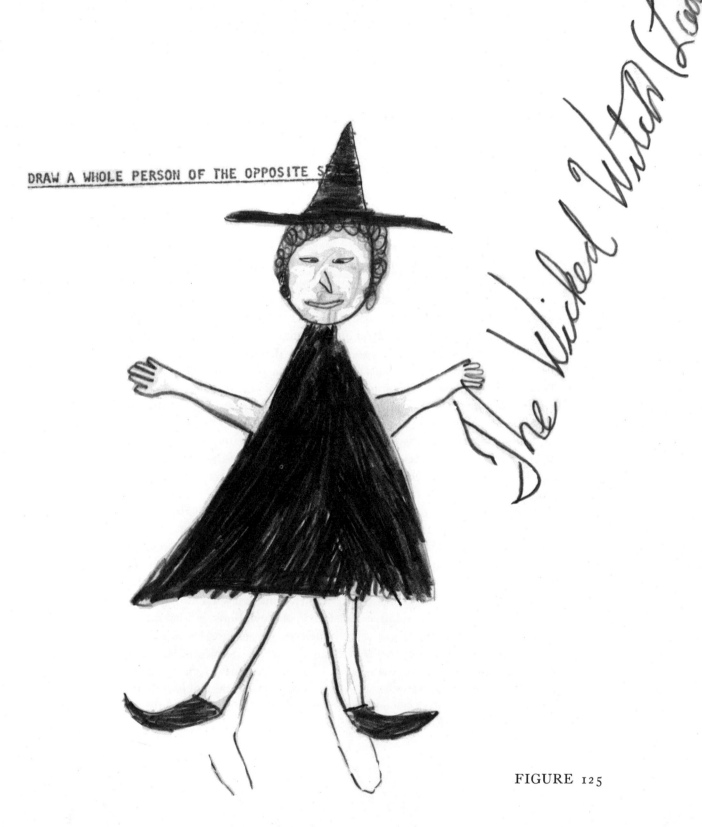

DRAW A WHOLE PERSON OF THE OPPOSITE S[...]

The Wicked Witch (Lady)

FIGURE 125

95

CHAPTER VIII

Psychosis

The human figure drawings of psychotic adolescents show enormous variety. This is clearly a reflection of the multi-faceted aspects of psychosis. These projected self-images must be viewed as symbols of a dynamic process, for as Bender states, "any picture or image is essentially a symbol, not a duplicate of what it represents." The highly disturbed individual attempts to redefine reality as he perceives it in terms of his own body ego. Thus, his distorted productions may be richly revealing of the nature of his fantasy life, as well as of the degree of fragmentation of his ego. The conflicts of the unconscious readily break through the weakened defensive structure of these patients and are often more easily and quickly communicated in drawings than in words. This is especially true of the young who are sometimes better able to reveal their attitudes towards the self and the significant others in their lives through the more concrete act of drawing than through abstract verbal ideation.

Time and again patients come to the clinic with complaints which represent only a protective facade. When they present us with a bizarre human figure drawing at the time of their very first visit, even the least sophisticated of our staff is alerted to the possibility of deeper underlying psychopathology. Heightened awareness of the examiner can then set the stage for more painstaking, sensitive interview techniques.

In contrast to the relative constancy of deviations in the human figure drawings of the organically impaired, we see great fluidity and change in those done by psychotic and borderline adolescents. These drawings, perhaps more than those of other patients, reflect the internal and external stresses they are currently experiencing. Their shattered, depreciated self-image, their fear of others, their confusion and hostility become instantly visible.

C.A.   *Age 12½ & 14*   *Male*   *I.Q. Above Average*

The patient suffers from restlessness and lack of concentration in school despite above average intelligence. He disrupts home life because of frequent fights with his sister and parents. He is underweight and undersized. He has no friends, attributing this to fear of being teased because of his small size. His frustration tolerance and impulse control are poor. He becomes overwhelmed by anger, then feels guilty. He turns anger and guilt against himself, resulting in bouts of depression.

He has been in psychiatric treatment at another clinic where the diagnosis of schizophrenia has been made on the basis of 1) poor object relations, 2) rage, 3) ego deficits, 4) pathological defense mechanisms.

Neurological examination and electroencephalogram are negative.

Drawings: The male looks like an inflated balloon simulating a clown. Concave mouth and buttons indicate dependency. Fin-like infantile outstretched short arms have only 4 fingers. No neck, no hair, undifferentiated trunk, no ears and no feet reveal marked maturational delay or ego regression. The eyes placed on the side of the head reveal a paranoid attitude. The figure appears to be floating in space.

The female figure is equally regressed but in a somewhat different manner. Instead of the inflated figure, we see a stick-like armature with a rudimentary skirt representing the trunk. Eyes are more centrally placed. Arms and hands are scribbled and undifferentiated. Balloon-like lower appendages represent undifferentiated legs and feet. Both drawings are essentially primitive and totally unrelated to the boy's intelligence.

(*Continued on next two pages.*)

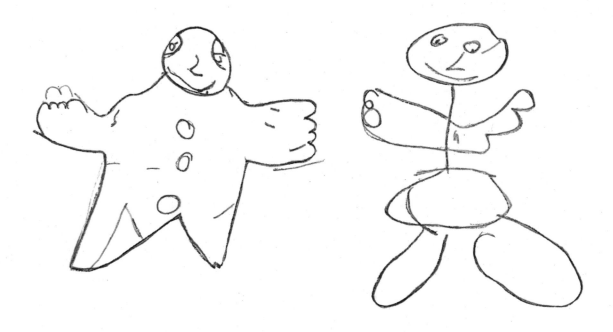

FIGURE 126   FIGURE 127

97

Fifteen months later we have another set of drawings (fiures 128 and 129) done by this patient, now 14 years old. Although he has made some progress, now offering hair, pupils, neck, breasts and legs, the essential bizarre "stupid" quality remains. The cross-hatching and wavy lines, the erasures, reenforcements and changes represent an increase in overt anxiety and a weak attempt to establish ego boundaries. The transparency of the female, with her global womb-like quality, reveals his infantile sexual preoccupation. The abortive, small, bird-like figure done in profile in the upper left hand corner of the page with the male drawing indicates his feeling of being sub-human. He is able to reject this projected concept and go on to a robot stage of man, still not quite human.

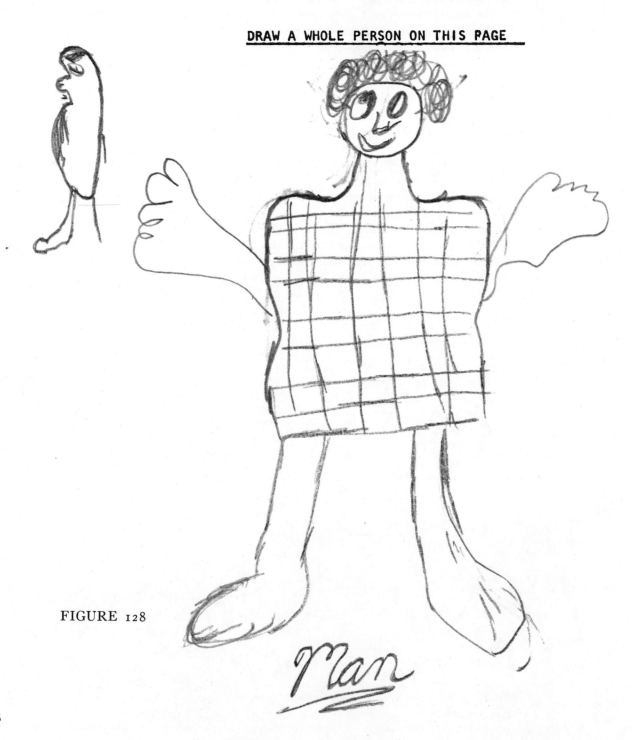

DRAW A WHOLE PERSON ON THIS PAGE

Man

FIGURE 128

98

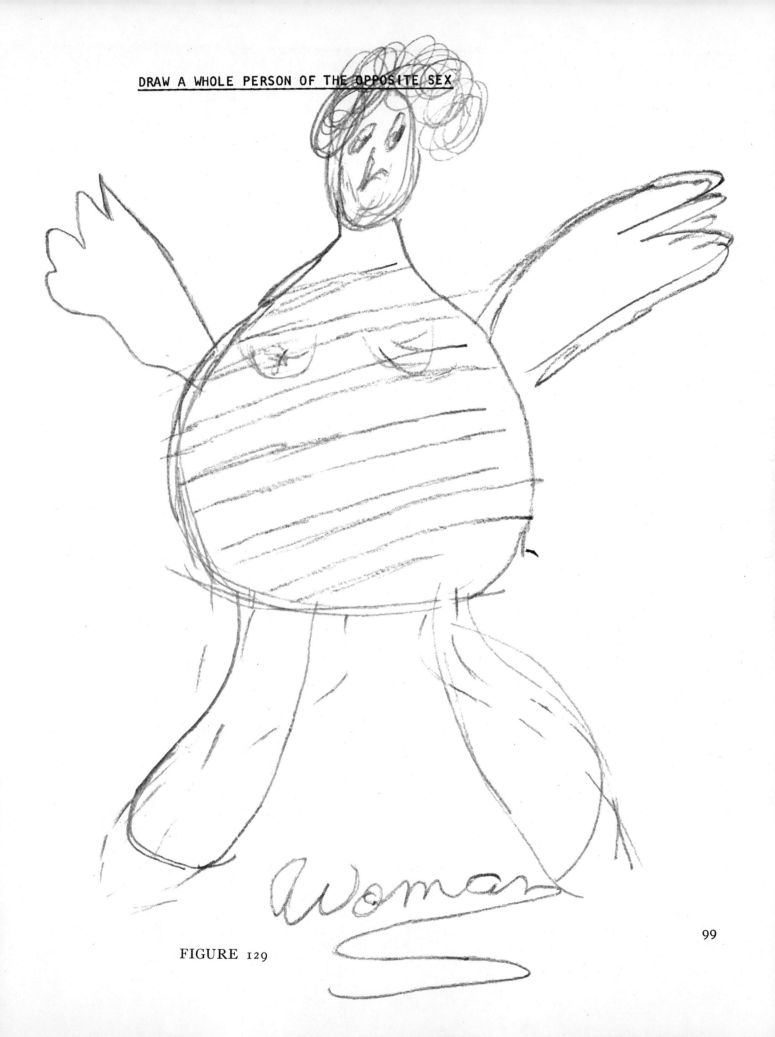

FIGURE 129

99

C.B.   Age 16   Male

This case is an excellent example of a patient who presents himself with simple somatic symptoms, headaches and fatigue, disguising serious psychopathology. In the first interview, his attitude was defiant, suspicious, withholding and hyper-intellectual. Restrained rage was palpable in his voice and manner as he discussed his father's multiple sclerosis, his mother's full-time job, his own social isolation and fear of impending school failure because of difficulty in concentration. The blame for his condition was projected onto others in typical paranoid fashion.

Drawings: Total disjunction of the body ego is experienced by this boy suffering from an acute paranoid schizophrenic reaction. He conceives of himself as a paper doll in separate sections.

He sees the female in profile and in action, well integrated but double-faced. He labels this "Picasso-esque," covering his fear and distrust of the girl with sly cleverness. The girl's head, skimpily indicating anxiety and uncertainty, also sports a small pointed beard. This upwardly displaced phallic projection aptly reveals his anxiety that the girl may indeed be more sexually powerful than he.

Two months later, somewhat improved on psychotropic medication, the patient drew a rigid but integrated male figure, joining the body parts together in a normal Gestalt (figure 132).

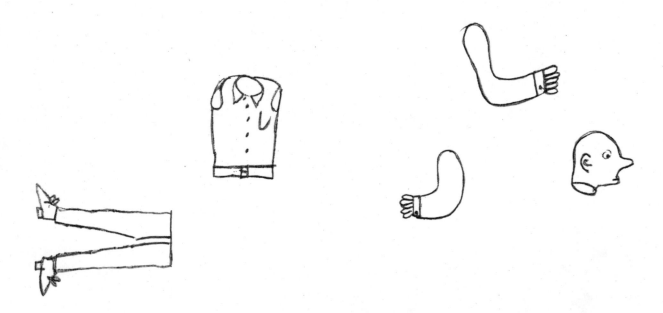

"The whole is the sum of its parts"
(Except in sub-atomic physics)

FIGURE 130

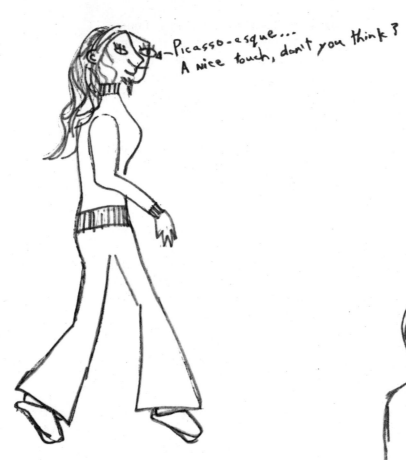

FIGURE 131

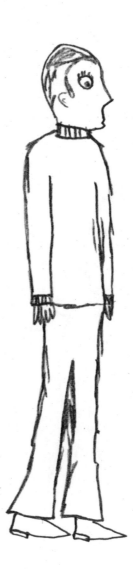

FIGURE 132

C.C.   *Age 15*   *Male*   *Low Average Intelligence*

The patient was referred by his school because of truancy, immature disruptive behavior, and lack of peer relationships. He was born with clubfeet and strabismus. Surgery for the latter at age 3 elicited from this child a state of extreme separation anxiety and clinging object relationships. His mother reacted to his demands by absenting herself from the home as much as possible and attempting to ignore his problems. His moods are labile, his impulse control is weak and he readily regresses under stress, even of a mild degree. He has difficulty organizing his thoughts, which are often infantile and illogical. One year ago he underwent surgery for an undescended testicle.

Drawings: Both figures are extremely primitive. The male head is that of a donkey, including the pointed ears. Interestingly, this boy who was born with strabismus puts a pupil only in the left eye. The wide gaping mouth indicates the enormity of his oral aggression. The body lacks all detail and has no genitality. Perhaps the recent orchopexy has intensified feelings of castration. The hands and feet are incapable of doing anything in their rudimentary state. The wavy lines indicate anxiety.

The female is smaller, poorly integrated and poorly executed. Her outstretched arms and crossed legs suggest a whirling movement. This is consonant with schizophrenic symptomatology, but may also reflect his feelings that his mother is always running, as indeed she is.

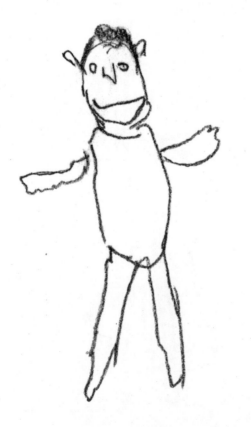

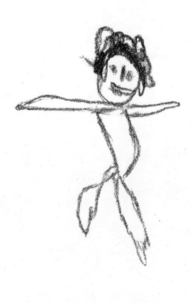

FIGURE 133   FIGURE 134

C.D.   *Age 12½*   *Female*   *Average Intelligence*

The patient was brought to the clinic by her parents because of obesity, lack of friends and extremely hostile behavior towards her father. Outside the home, she is excessively conforming and peculiarly naive. Her father often walks about the house unclothed, enraging the patient.

In the interview the patient had a bland facade, but quickly broke into tears. Psychological testing revealed wide intra-test scatter, with a performance I.Q. of 83 and a verbal I.Q. of 115. She revealed phobic and paranoid ideation, constriction, anxiety and a negative self-image.

Drawings: Both sexes are drawn as virtually identical stick figures without faces. Aggressive spokes protrude from the heads. Fists reach out threateningly from these primitive sub-human figures.

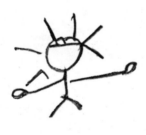

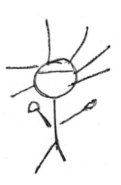

FIGURE 135   FIGURE 136

FIGURES 137, 138

C.E.   *Age 12½*   *Male*   *I.Q. 91*

The patient was admitted to the hospital for diagnosis of abdominal pain of 6 weeks duration. The clinical and laboratory findings revealed a mild viral infection from which he was almost fully recovered. However, his complaints continued and he was reluctant to return to school. Investigation revealed that he was a highly dependent boy, scapegoated by his peers because of a speech impediment and ungainly appearance. Psychological testing revealed bizarre fantasies, weak defenses and poor reality testing.

Drawings: Both figures have a bizarre quality and transparencies consistent with poor reality testing. The male nose is markedly phallic, while the pelvic areas are a mass of confused lines and erasures. He cannot decide whether or not the legs start at the waist. The huge male head placed on a thin neck symbolizes obsessional ideation and isolation of affect corroborated by projective test findings. The spindly, low-slung arms of the boy terminate in outstretched aggressive hands with pronounced knuckles and nails.

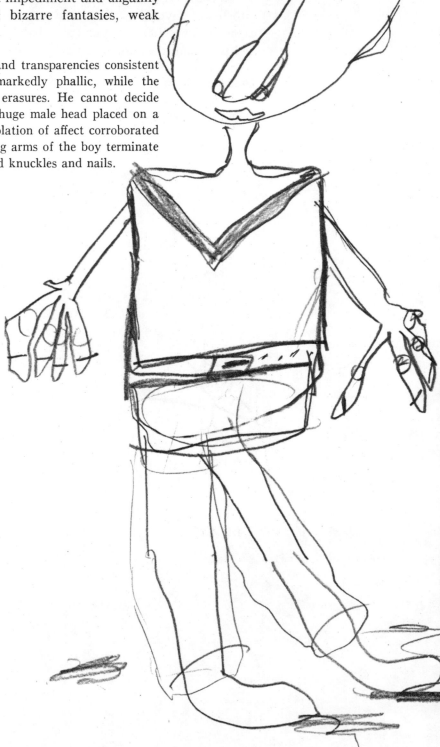

FIGURE 137

104

The drawing of the female was intended as a portrait of the pregnant psychologist. He asked many inappropriate anxious questions about pregnancy such as, "Are maternity clothes made of special bloodproof material?" As the scribbled whorls burst out of the abdomen, so did he seem to fearfully anticipate that the baby might be born any minute, right then and there.

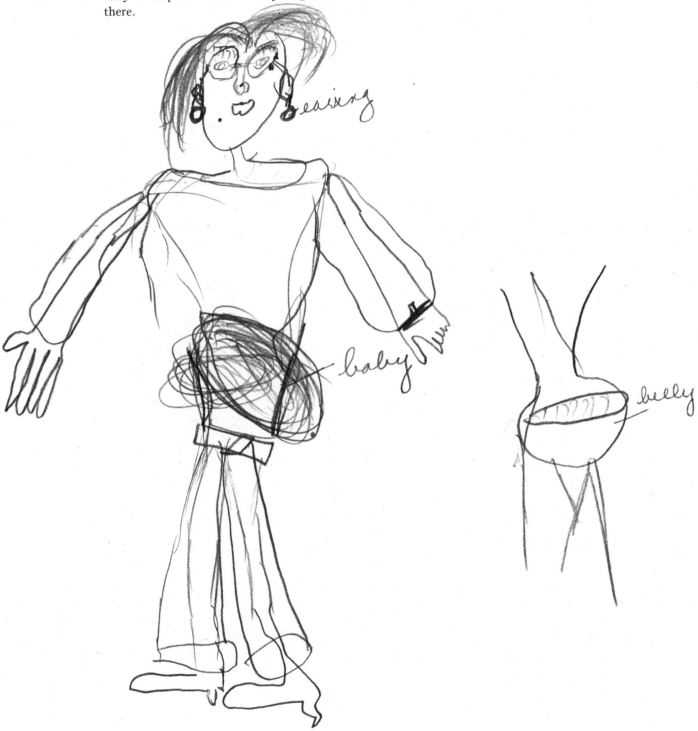

FIGURE 138

C.F.   *Age 19*   *Male*

This reluctant patient was brought to the clinic by his mother for a "total" evaluation. He had suffered a "nervous breakdown" a year earlier and refused to continue in psychiatric treatment after a brief attempt, fearing that he would be considered "crazy." Investigation revealed that he had been brought up symbiotically by his mother who had never permitted the youth any independent action or decisions. His only success has been in the academic area. His sad and lonely life is preoccupied with autistic fantasies.

Drawings: Although sad and empty, these figure drawings are not as pathological as other projective tests in this case. Intellectual and compulsive defenses help to keep him in check. The uneven arms lack hands, rendering them impotent. The broken outlines indicate anxiety. The breasts of the female represent the patient's need for nurturing rather than sex, as his psychosexual development is fixated at the oral-anal level. The midline emphasis of the girl's skirt shows preoccupation with this "forbidden" area. The relatively small size of the heads suggests a wish to rid himself of troublesome thoughts.

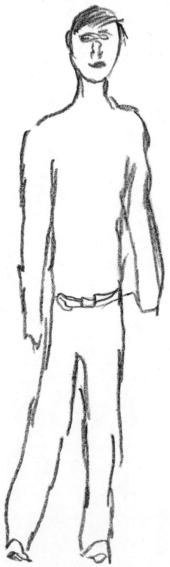

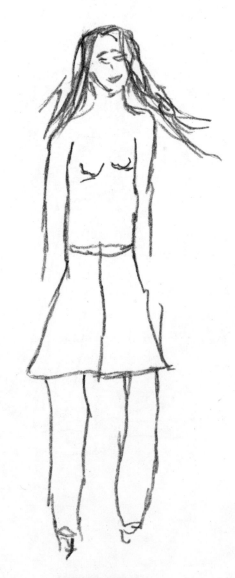

106

FIGURE 139   FIGURE 140

C.G.   *Age 13*   *Female*

The patient was brought to the clinic by her mother because of behavior problems and obesity. The latter condition developed following her father's death two years earlier, for which she felt responsible. She claims to dearly love her older brother who has "replaced father," but feels that he hates her. She has been truanting and failing the school year. When a routine blood test was to be done in the clinic, the patient went into a state of panic.

Drawings: Both figures are grossly immature and bizarre. It is evident from the wide spread between the girl's curved stick legs and the boy's gigantic penis that she is obsessed with incestuous fantasies. This explains her inordinate sense of guilt and psychic disorganization. She has displaced oedipal longing for her father onto her brother. The clublike, undifferentiated hands and feet indicate intense aggression and impulsive acting out. The drawings lack necks and are poorly integrated in all respects.

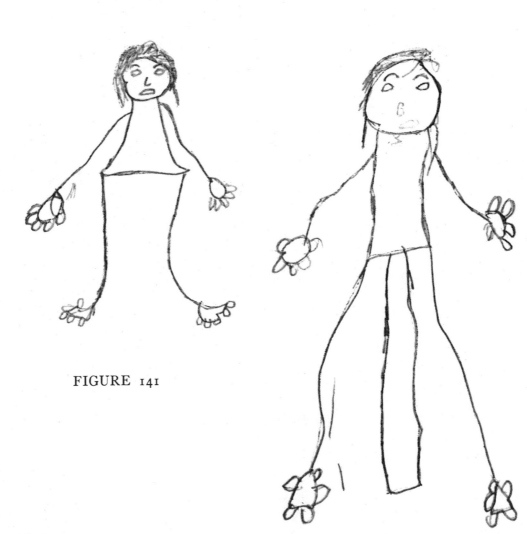

FIGURE 141

FIGURE 142

C.I.   *Age 13*   *Male*   *I.Q. 73*

This patient was brought to the clinic by his mother with a multitude of complaints and an unusual history. He complained of headaches, nausea and dizziness of 6 months duration. He is very highstrung, stutters, bites his nails and cries easily. A younger brother is epileptic and has received most of the mother's attention.

The mother dates the patient's stuttering back to age 5, when a traumatic incident occurred which was never mentioned until the day of this interview. The boy was waiting in a car for his grandfather who was shopping. When the grandfather returned to the car after a few minutes, the boy was gone. He arrived home three hours later in a distraught state, babbling about "a man." The family felt that he had been "kidnapped," perhaps even molested, and chose to bury the matter. When he entered school, he was unable to learn and showed no curiosity. This is often the case where there has been a conspiracy of silence and significant material is repressed. Repeated school failure reenforced the boy's image of himself as stupid. He developed a de-

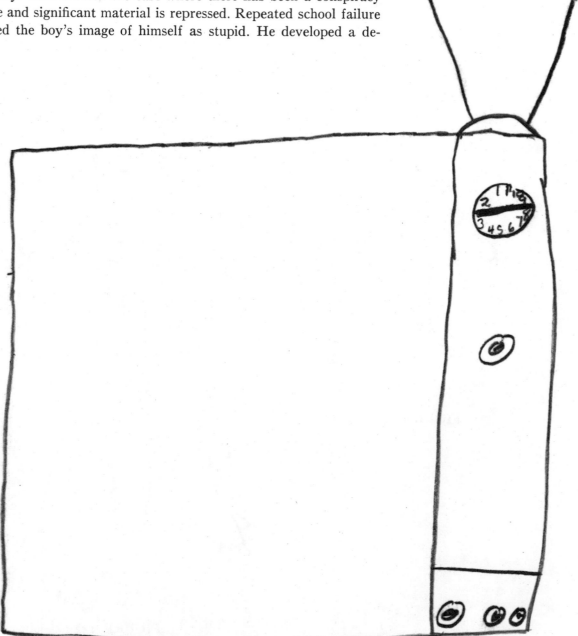

FIGURE 143

fensive pleasant smile and blandness, belied by his many symptoms.

The borderline I.Q. he obtained is an average based on wide intra-test scatter, a finding consonant with his severe emotional problems. Equivocal organic signs on psychological testing further confused the diagnostic picture.

Drawings: The diagnosis is clarified by these startling productions. The patient sees himself as depersonalized, a kind of grandfather (see history above) clock with numbers reversed and antennae reaching out. The detached pendulum disc suggests an umbilicus. The second drawing is his very own disembodied face, an uncanny resemblance! These are certainly not the drawings of a retarded adolescent. They do, however, support the diagnosis of pseudo-retarded childhood schizophrenia.

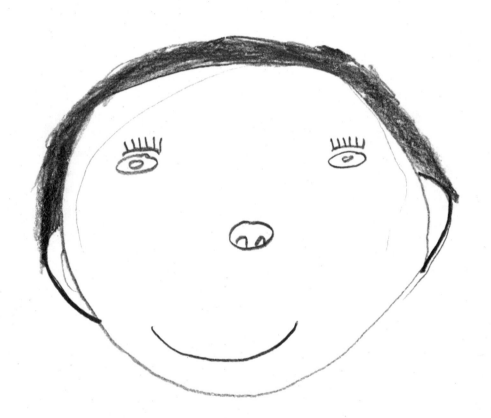

FIGURE 144

C.H.   Age 15   Male   I.Q. 114

The school complains that he torments his peers, constantly seeks attention and cannot maintain interest in his work. These difficulties have existed since early childhood. He teases his siblings and is otherwise troublesome at home. The patient denies having any problems!

Drawings: The figures are bizarre robots, silly and aggressive at the same time. The male wears a crown suggesting grandiose aspirations for power, while totally lacking a pelvis. There are numerous anatomical omissions. The double lines at shoulder and waist represent an attempt at compulsive controls. The out-turned large feet signify poor impulse control.

The female also has a wide, transparent space between her legs. Perhaps the patient's fantasy is that she has a cloaca. The perseverative circles representing buttons, knees, etc. are further symbols of infantile sexuality.

These drawings, in a boy with an I.Q. of 114, strongly suggest psychosis.

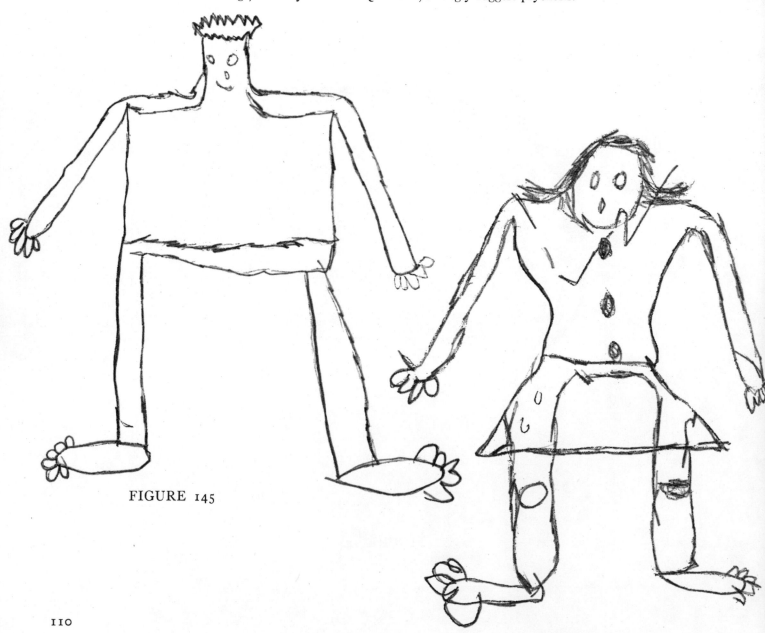

FIGURE 145

FIGURE 146

C.J.   *Age 13*   *Male*   *I.Q. 100*

The patient has always done poorly in school, does no work and has only girls as friends. He was operated on three times for strabismus before the age of 6. He uses only one eye and tilts his head to the right to see. This gives him an odd appearance of which he is conscious. He is infantilized by his mother and overshadowed by a younger, more capable brother. He has grown increasingly withdrawn, inhibited and apathetic since the onset of adolescence.

Drawings: These primitive, pin-headed, sausage figures are differentiated only by the presence of more hair on the girl's head. The absence of arms and hands, among other things, render these "people" totally incapable. The toed-in feet make them pathetically crippled. With a self-image such as this, it is small wonder that the boy has given up trying.

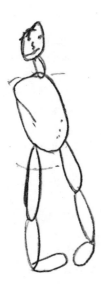

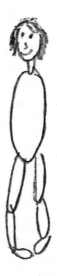

FIGURE 147   FIGURE 148

CHAPTER IX

Danger Signals: Acting-Out, Suicide and Homicide

Adolescence has been regarded as a time when at least some degree of impulsive, rebellious or assertive behavior is expected. Common time-worn expressions such as "sowing his wild oats" reveal the expectation of strongly emerging drives and behavior which expresses these drives. Early adolescence is a period in which quiescent sexual and aggressive fantasies and impulses reemerge, gaining momentum and strength. The individual during his adolescent years must learn to integrate these drives and find socially acceptable ways of expressing them and obtain or defer satisfactions for the tensions they generate. At the same time, the adolescent is trying to assert his independence and find an identity separate from that of his parents and family. Thus, there are several factors operating which would make experimentation and acting-out a normal stage of development. Usually this behavior does not take forms which are dangerous to the teenager or to those around him. When the adolescent's behavior is interpreted as abnormal, intolerable or dangerous by adults, he is brought to the attention of the professional. Often the perception of his behavior is subjective and colored by many factors.

One form of acting-out is overt expression of sexual drive through pre-marital sexual activity. Sanctions against such activity, interpretations of "bad" and "destructive" are largely determined by the culture and the sex of the teenager. In many groups a boy is encouraged and applauded for his sexual encounters, whereas a girl is strongly castigated. Even physical expression of aggression has a heavy cultural determinant in its acceptability. Wrestling and fist fighting, or expressions of manliness through minor delinquent acts, serve as a "rite de passage" among many groups in our society. Where physical violence of any type is deplored, such behavior would be interpreted as disruptive and alarming.

Undesirable acting-out behavior can include verbal aggression toward authority figures, neglect of school work, truanting, running away, sexual promiscuity, violent attacks upon people and property, and self-destructive acts such as drug abuse and suicidal attempts. The question asked the professional is whether acting-out behavior toward others or oneself is likely to occur or recur. The rising rate of adolescent suicide and homicide makes detection of such tendencies an issue of paramount importance. It is the practitioner's responsibility to make assessments of impulse control and, when possible, predict acting-out tendencies before the overt act is committed. In the following selected human figure drawings, the individual's potential for acting-out, as well as his controls against these impulses, is illustrated.

FIGURE 149

H.A.   *Age 13*   *Male*

The patient was referred for psychological evaluation by Children's Court, after he was charged with assaulting a teacher.

Drawing: The general character of the drawing is rather empty, with little detail given to the face. The stance is typical of the rebellious, evasive teenager, with face in profile, jutting jaw and blank eye. The posture suggests lunging or jumping. The pointed feet and broadened hands indicate acting-out potential. The head is not connected to the body, reflecting difficulties with impulse control. The flattened head raises the question of an organic component in the behavior. The affect of the drawing is angry and aggressive.

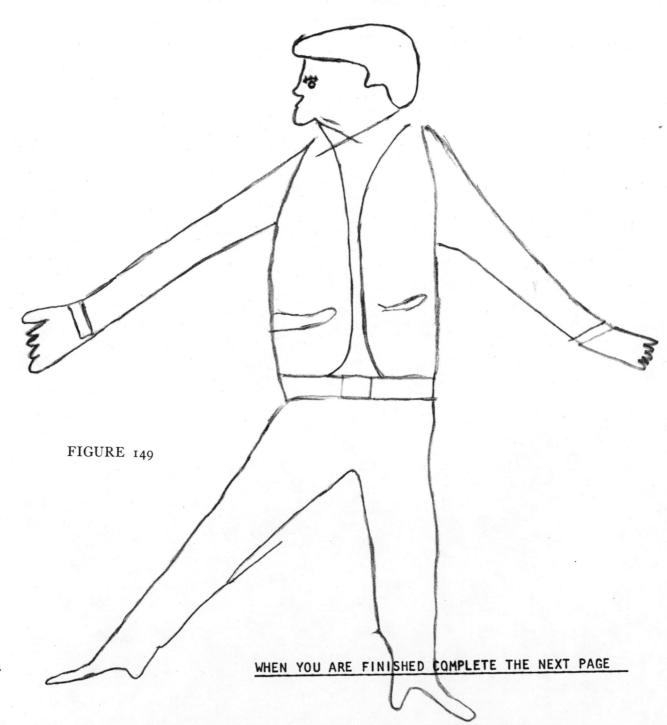

FIGURE 149

WHEN YOU ARE FINISHED COMPLETE THE NEXT PAGE

FIGURE 150

H.B.   *Age 14*   *Male*

This youngster presents many behavior problems, including temper tantrums, verbal abuse of teachers, inability to relate to peers and stealing. He is reported to be likable and amenable to direction in a one-to-one situation with an adult. His parents are divorced and mother is very rejecting. She refuses to obtain psychiatric help for the boy.

Drawing: The figure is designated "girl," yet is extremely ambiguous in sexual identification. This is quite unusual as boys of 14 are generally well defended against conscious bisexual fantasies. The eyes are closed both in a seductive gesture and in an effort to guard against what might be seen. This could be defensive reaction-formation against voyeurism directed towards his mother, with whom he lives alone. Although shading and compulsive striping are common at this age, they are unusually placed in this case. Great feelings of anger and hostility are evident in the fingers and darkened pointed nails. Shading over the shoulder and upper arm and striping of the lower arm symbolize a wish to maintain some control over expression of these feelings. Collar and buttons on the neck are a further attempt at constricting his hostility.

FIGURE 150

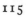

THIS IS A Girl

FIGURE 151

H.C.   *Age 14*   *Male*

This boy was referred for evaluation because of disruptive class-room behavior and academic failure.

Drawing: The open truncation of the arms and legs indicates fluidity in body boundaries. The absence of hands reflects difficulty in making inter-personal contact. The missing feet are indicative of an inability to stand up independently. A side profile generally indicates both evasiveness and rebelliousness. The emphasized eye and ear are signs of suspiciousness. The absence of lines separating head, neck and body is a predictor of acting-out tendency, as the neck is considered to be the control area between intellect and impulse.

FIGURE 151

FIGURE 152

H.D.   *Age 13*   *Male*

This boy is involved in numerous classroom fights with students and verbal altercations with teachers.

Drawing: The figure is propelled from without by a rocket and suspended in mid-air, indicating difficulty in controlling impulses. A fusion of sexual and aggressive impulses is reflected in the rocket, the projection on top of the rocket, and fire covering the lower part of the body. The absent controls are obvious in the neckless body and the featureless face. The open mouth is suggestive of orality aggressively expressed.

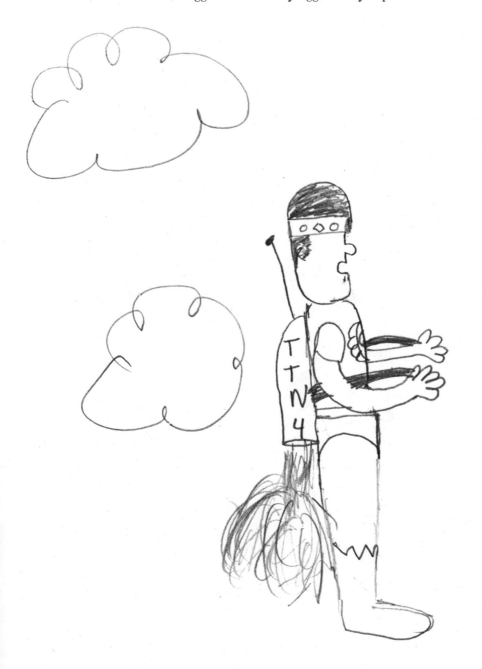
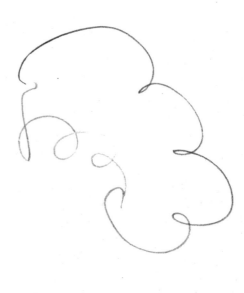

FIGURE 152

FIGURE 153

H.E.   *Age 15*   *Male*

Patient jumped off a Long Island Railroad train because he was afraid that police would arrest him for riding on the roof. He sustained a skull fracture and was brought to the hospital.

Drawing: Both body image and defenses are relatively intact. The stance and the facial expression convey the message of being ready to fight. In an otherwise well proportioned drawing, the arms are unusually long and the hands are excessively large. The broad shoulders and clenched fist add to the impression of an acting out potential. One gets the feeling of anger barely restrained by obsessive-compulsive defenses. The clenched fists protruding from tightly buttoned cuffs and the detailed palm lines reveal an effort to control his aggression. The pointed feet are also acting-out indicators. The very idealized masculine aspect of the figure gives the impression that the patient has a strong need to prove his masculinity and might do so by engaging in reckless pursuits.

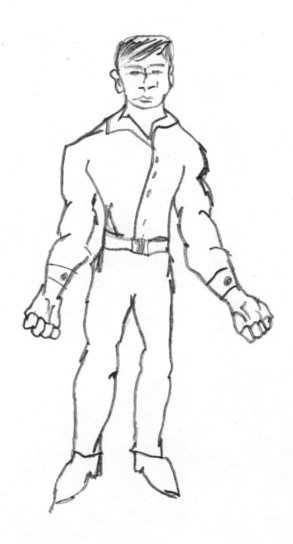

FIGURE 153

FIGURE 154

H.F.   *Age 17*   *Male*

The patient is a diabetic boy who attends boarding school because of his inability to get along with his family. He uses various drugs including hashish, LSD and mescaline.

Drawing: The subject depicted is a stereotype of the "in" teenager. However, several unusual features appear which differentiate this drawing from typical ones. Although a guitar is not an uncommon item in this age group, this is the only electric one with connection to an amplifier. A dependence on being "turned on" in order to be heard is implied. The foot on the box is a common element in the drawings of several acting-out youngsters, indicating insecurity. This patient's feeling of inferiority, intensified by his reliance on insulin, causes him to use drugs to achieve some sense of adequacy.

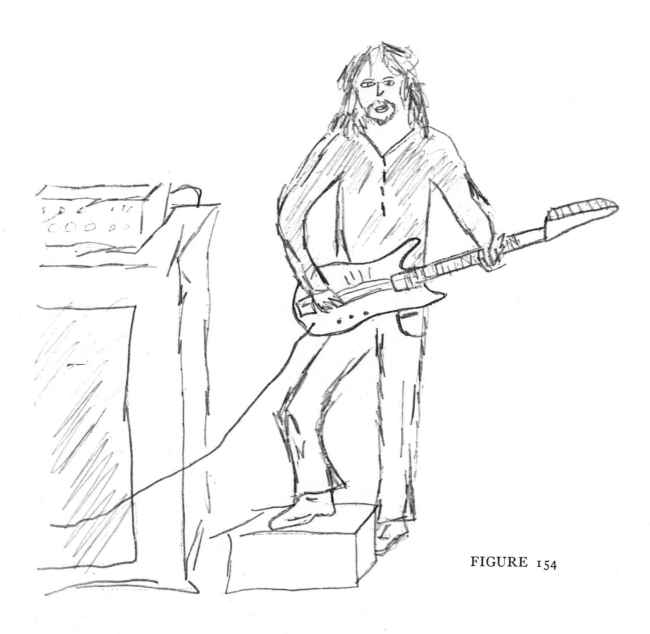

FIGURE 154

FIGURE 155

H.G.   Age 18   Male   Average Intelligence

The patient has marked growth retardation and a 6-year history of heroin addiction. He supports the habit by shoplifting when necessary. He was hospitalized for study of his growth failure, but walked out before discharge, presumably because of his need for heroin.

Drawing: Acting-out tendency is inferred by omission. An impaired ego and absent defenses may be inferred from the empty, regressed state of the figure. The absence of neck and hands indicates lack of control over his aggressive impulses. The face is expressionless, the eyes and mouth fixed, completely closed to contact with the world. Such an individual is likely to seek gratification and reduction of tension at all cost.

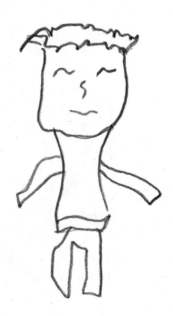

FIGURE 155

FIGURE 156

H.H.   *Age 17*   *Male*

The patient came to the clinic for the treatment of ophthalmological symptoms. He is a poor student and has been on marijuana and heroin.

Drawing: Although the patient has adequate artistic ability, this is a poor drawing. Tension is indicated in the shaky line quality. The general impression of a poor sense of body integrity is striking. The chest area is overemphasized, probably because of somatic preoccupation. Most marked is the angry, unhappy facial expression, with a heavily emphasized mouth showing much oral need and concern. There is little in the drawing to indicate defenses against acting-out, and if oral gratification is desperately needed (drugs), behavior is likely to be geared to this end.

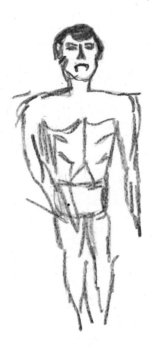

FIGURE 156

FIGURES 157, 158

H.J.   *Age 17*   *Female*

The patient has a 2-year history of heroin addiction, for which she was hospitalized. Her current complaint is hepatitis.

Drawings: The detailing and good proportion of the drawing indicate a superior artist, above average in intelligence. Psychosexual development in a 17-year-old should be at a stage of strong feminine identification. The choice of a male for the first drawing, the type of male depicted and the contrast in detailing between the male and female drawings preclude a feminine position. The male is essentially bisexual, attired in a skirt, with his hand held in an effeminate position. There are many phallic preoccupations as seen in the heavy shading in the thigh area, the dagger and spear. The profile view is rebellious. The open mouths seek oral gratification. The female is rather seductive in posture and attire, yet the cape suggests a disguise. Acting-out may occur in the form of oral gratification through drug use, sexual promiscuity as a defense against homosexuality, or aggressive anti-social behavior as an affirmation of having a fantasied phallus.

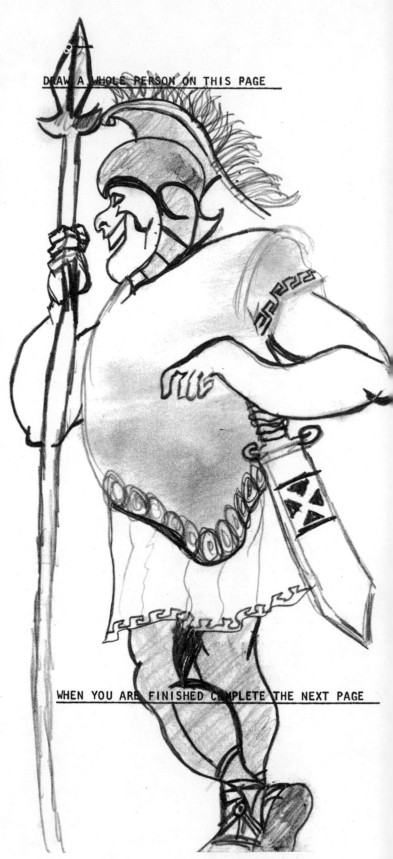

FIGURE 157

122

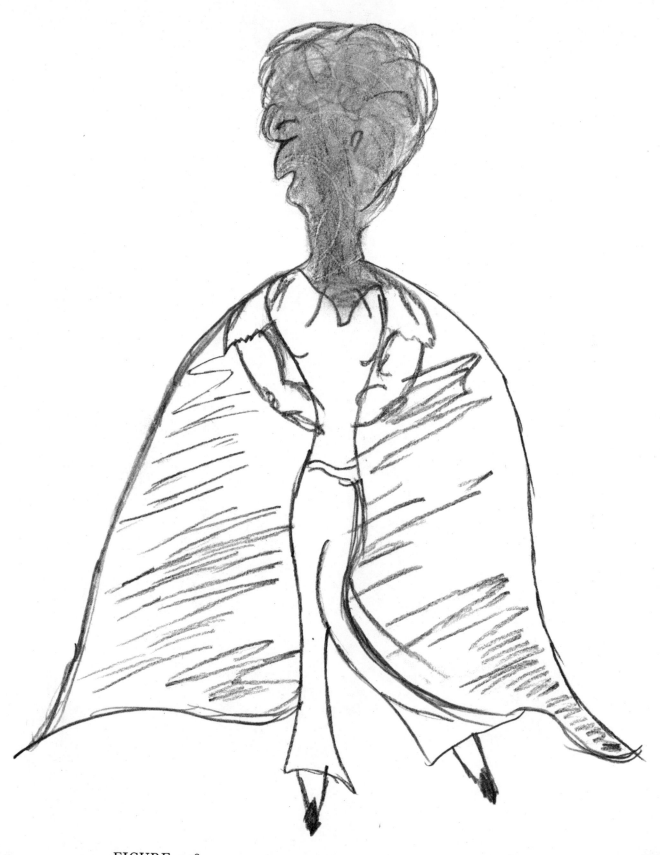

FIGURE 158

FIGURE 159

H.I.   *Age 14*   *Female*

This girl has been involved in heavy drug use, including heroin.

Drawing: The total impression is one of being out of control. The hair hangs down wildly and the facial expression is aggressive. The sharply opposed thumbs are an indicator of sexual preoccupation, probably on the masturbatory level. Poor impulse control is evident in the fusion of the head and body. Efforts to control aggressive impulses are weak and appear as a shaded band where the neck should be, and in the stripes on the left arm. Dependency ties are very strong as noted in the long cords dangling from the belt buckle. The open mouth indicates her great need for oral gratification. In adolescent girls, the stronger the regressive pull back to the mother, the greater the potential for acting-out behavior. Strong dependency, orality, and concomitant weak impulse control are indices of a high risk for drug abuse.

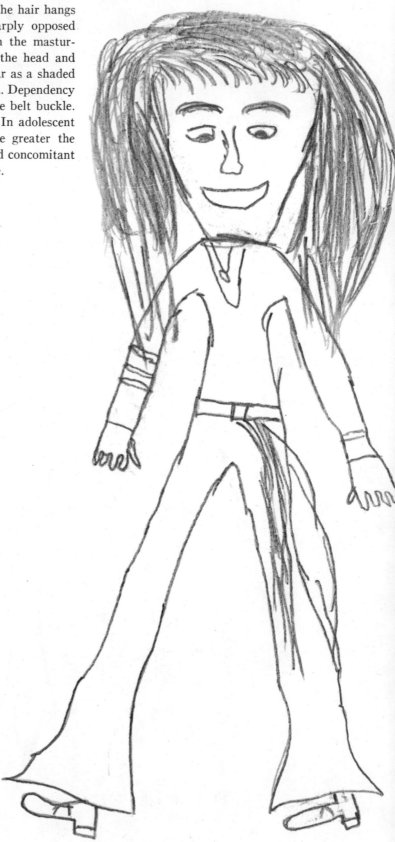

FIGURE 159

FIGURE 160

H.K.   *Age 18*   *Female*

This girl came to the emergency room complaining of dizziness. She had been living in a public park for two months, involved in drugs and prostitution.

Drawing: The figure represents the fantasy of a belly dancer. The dress, eyes and hair attempt to look seductive; yet the bulky, massive, unattractive body reflects the patient's negative self-image. Although the navel is revealed in such a costume, its inclusion, as well as the infantile bud mouth, reflects great dependency upon the mother. The short, ineffectual arms terminate in pointed, hostile fingers. The scrolls covering the costume indicate the girl's maze-like confusion about acting out her bodily impulses. Generally, the figure lacks feminine identification, and is indicative of a girl who has not reached a stage of adult heterosexuality. Acting-out behavior may be a defense against her weak feminine identification.

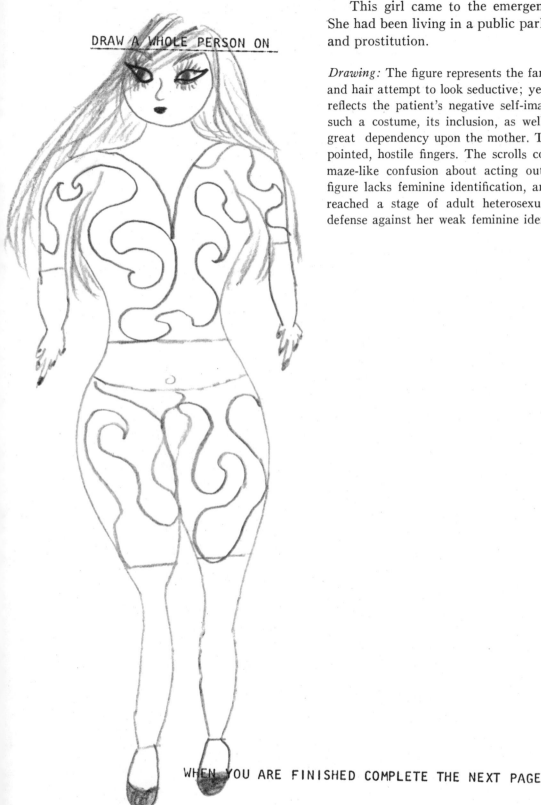

DRAW A WHOLE PERSON ON

WHEN YOU ARE FINISHED COMPLETE THE NEXT PAGE

FIGURE 160   125

FIGURE 161

H.L.   *Age 16*   *Male*

The patient suffers from depression, lack of interest in school and conflict with his parents. He failed to keep several appointments for psychiatric evaluation. On his first visit, a thought disorder was evident.

Drawing: The general quality of the drawing is fragmented. The body is amorphous and incomplete. The arms are indistinct and the hands and feet absent, indicating inability to make contact with others and lack of mobility. The vagueness of the outlines and poor definition of body parts reflect depersonalization and personality disintegration. The multiple slashes in the arms and chest and the halo-like slash through the head indicate his wish to harm himself physically. This patient should be regarded as a high risk for a self-destructive act.

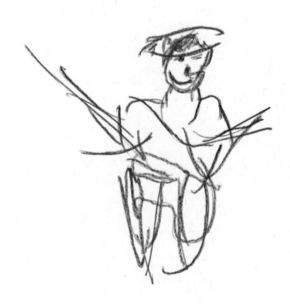

FIGURE 161

FIGURE 162

H.M.   *Age 19*   *Male College Graduate*

The patient was admitted to the hospital following an overdose. He was subsequently treated in an outpatient psychiatric clinic. Ten months after this human figure drawing was done, the patient committed suicide.

Drawing: The general body form and line quality are poor. There is a feeling of disintegration in the whole body image, which reflects the patient's failing defenses. The selection of a female as the first figure drawn in a 19-year-old male is unusual and indicative of confusion in sexual identification. Explicit detailing of breasts, especially in the absence of other sexual organs, shows fixation or regression to an oral dependent state. This is substantiated by the heavily outlined concave mouth. The dark dots in the ear area indicate aural preoccupation, probably caused by auditory hallucinations. A strong acting-out tendency is revealed in the excessively long, broadened arms with wide spreading fingers. By contrast, the sharply truncated thumbs point up feelings of castration. On the lower left side of the body, extending through the left thigh to the midline, is a pencil slash. Although this type of line looks accidental, its recurrent presence in the drawings of suicidal patients has given it the name of "suicidal slash."

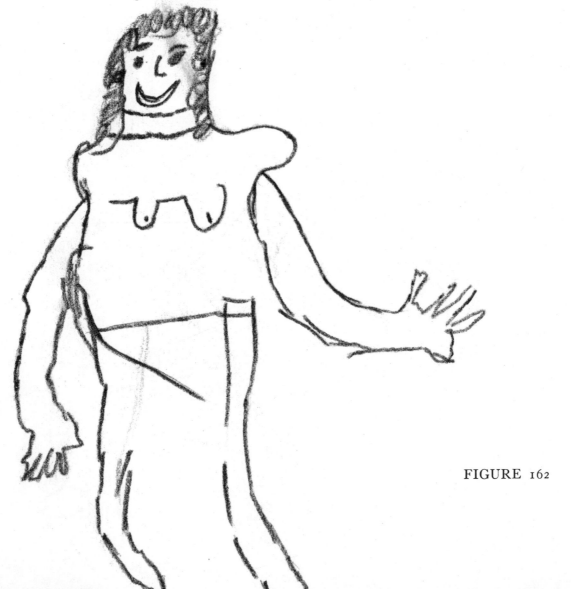

FIGURE 162

H.N. *Age 15* *Female*

This girl was admitted to the adolescent service suffering from a gastric ulcer which was successfully treated with diet and medication. Shortly after her discharge, she made a suicide attempt and was admitted to the psychiatric ward. The drawings were obtained two days apart, the second one half an hour after the patient slashed her wrist superficially.

Drawings: The faces have a plaintive, childlike quality. The marked slant of the figures reflects the girl's feeling of being off-balance emotionally. The slash on the lower torso and leg area of the second drawing is indicative of the girl's wish to harm herself.

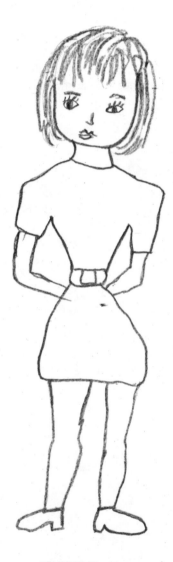

FIGURE 163

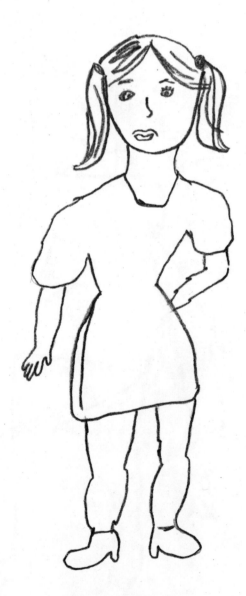

FIGURE 164

FIGURE 165

H.O.   *Age 16*   *Female*

This patient was admitted to the adolescent service after ingesting a near fatal dose of Doriden in a suicide attempt.

Drawing: The infantile quality, empty face, poor body proportion, absence of neck and displacement of arms to waist level are all indicative of neurological impairment. Since there is no previous evidence of organicity, the drawing may reflect the transient effects of drug overdosage. The dark circular slash in the chest and neck area is a suicide slash of particular significance because of its placement in a vital area of the body. This adolescent has serious intentions of committing suicide.

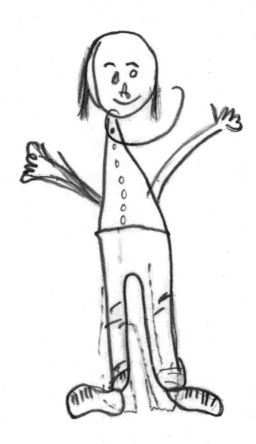

FIGURE 165

CHAPTER X

Follow-Up

We embarked on a limited random follow-up study, requesting patients to repeat the same task: *"Draw a Whole Person"* and then *"Draw a Person of the Opposite Sex."* The time interval was approximately 2 to 3 years. Our findings corroborate the indisputable fact that adolescence is a time of fluid change, both in ego maturation and in the shifting of defense mechanisms. The greater the psychopathology, the more fixated the patient and the less change is to be anticipated in the human figure drawings. The adolescent who is moving towards an adult adaptation to life becomes less inhibited, more imaginative, more certain of his sexual identification. The following examples demonstrate a wide variety of alterations in body representation, as well as some frozen in their earlier stage.

I.A.   *Age 15 & 16½*   *Female*

The patient came to the clinic for the treatment of moderate obesity. She lost weight and regained it.

Drawings: At 15 she drew a male first, immature and devoid of detail. The girl is more attractive than the boy, with more attention given to clothes and hair. The gaping open mouth is the only clue to her overeating problem. The body image is a wishful one.

One and a half years later, her drawings are done much more skillfully and compulsively. They are still idealized images, youth culture oriented. Although attractive, they are "tight" figures. Mouths are still prominent. The tight lacings, buttons and belts are stylish, but they also project the erection of compulsive defenses to ward off forbidden impulses. The line technique is much more assured. The girl is drawn first, signifying more acceptance of her feminine role. The character of the mouth remains unchanged.

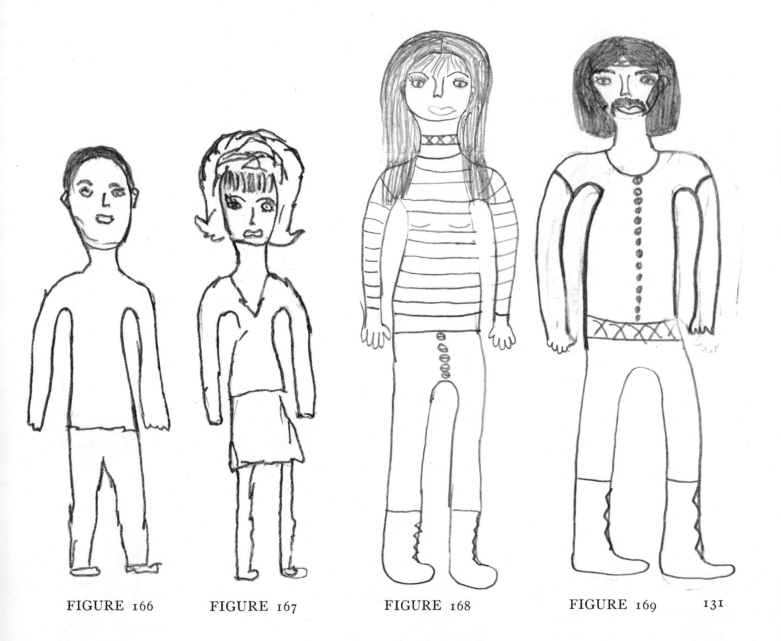

FIGURE 166   FIGURE 167   FIGURE 168   FIGURE 169   131

I.B.   Age 16 & 19   Female

This patient came for help because of chronic severe atopic eczema. The emotional climate in the home is an unhappy one because of the mother's expressed dissatisfaction with her marriage. There is also concern about a younger brother who is truanting and is attracted to delinquent friends. The patient herself is an academic over-achiever. In the three year interval between drawings, she attended and dropped out of an Ivy League college. She also solved some inner conflicts, as her drawings demonstrate.

Drawings: They are fascinating from two points of view, sexual and cultural. At 16, this serious-minded, middle-class black girl sees herself as nun-like, pure and aloof. Only the rippled hem of the cape implies the underlying sexual excitement which she is trying so hard to suppress. She sees the handsome Negro youth humbled to his knees, with his hands behind his back. In point of fact, the men in her family are passive.

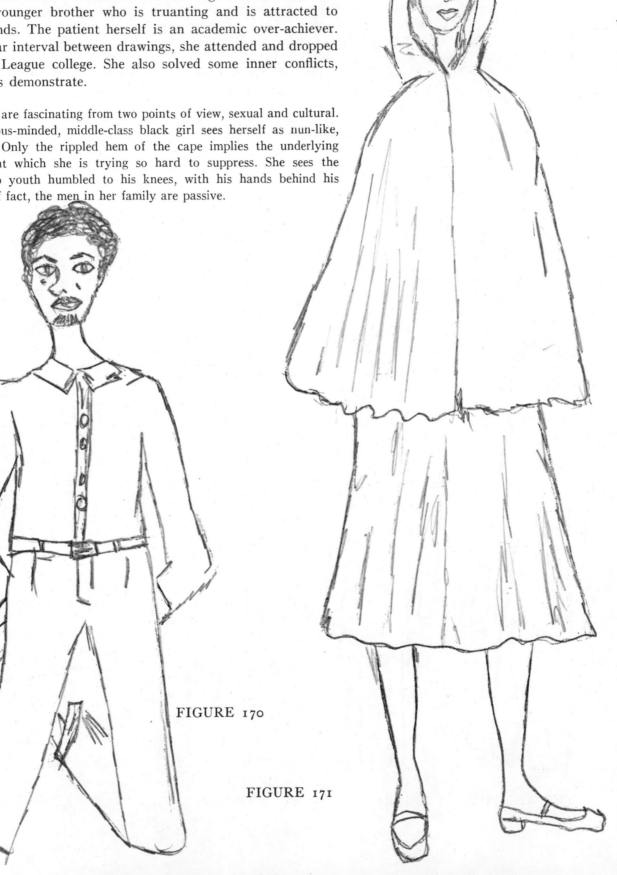

FIGURE 170

132

FIGURE 171

At 19, she sees "herself" as fashionably mini-skirted and bangled, self-confidently smiling. She is in a dancing posture. The well-drawn handsome male, wearing a dashiki, stands in a self-confident position with arms crossed. In the 3-year interval one feels that she has lost her rigid inhibitions and has found a sense of highly satisfying racial identification. In both sets of drawings, she did the male first. This is not unusual in an adolescent girl seeking a male partner.

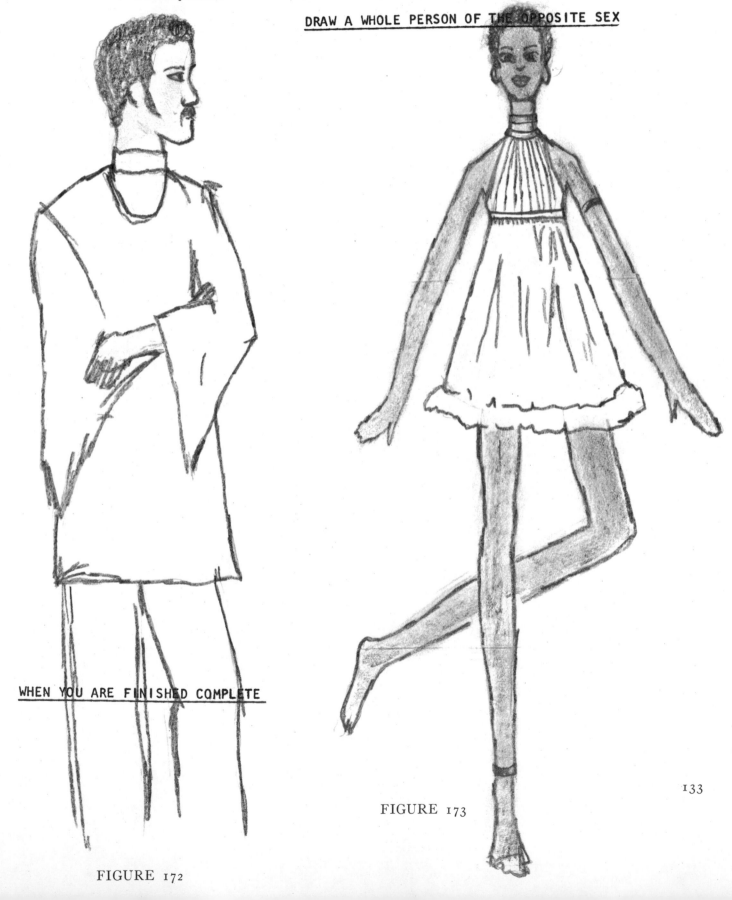

DRAW A WHOLE PERSON OF THE OPPOSITE SEX

WHEN YOU ARE FINISHED COMPLETE

FIGURE 172

FIGURE 173

133

I.C.   *Age 13 & 16*   *Female*

This patient came to the clinic for the treatment of widespread chronic eczema. She is an adopted only child, tightly controlled by her mother. She stutters, has nervous mannerisms and works very hard in school. When away from home, she is much more relaxed.

Drawings: At 13 she did not feel human. She perceived people as an odd combination of triangles, squares and lines. The figures resemble those done by brain-injured children. The girl's left hand, dangling from a single-line arm, has 6 fingers. The boundary lines are broken and uncertain, revealing her intense anxiety. The small head and long neck are seen in obsessional neurotics who would like to do less thinking. Obviously, this immature girl does not feel in touch with her own body, possibly disowning it because of the tormenting eczema she suffers. The male figure lacks a pelvis and shows even more anxiety in its execution.

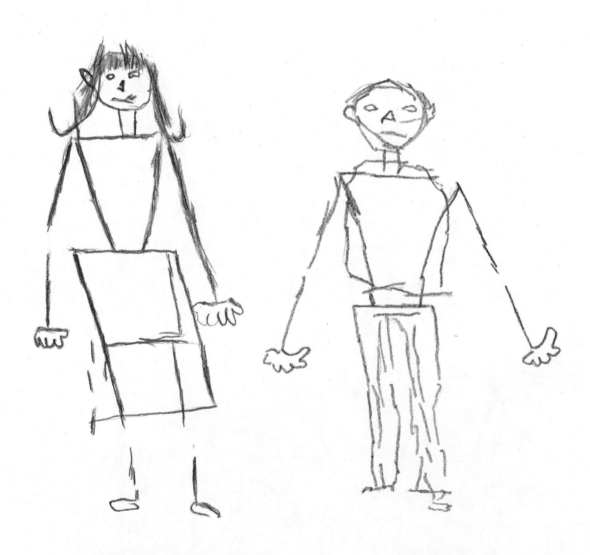

FIGURE 174   FIGURE 175

At 16 her human figure drawings are still grossly immature but humanized. It is as though she had to catch up on earlier developmental stages that were missed. The large head and single-line smiling mouth are typical of much younger children. The noses, previously drawn as simple triangles, are now quite phallic. The midline emphasis on the girl's torso shows somatic preoccupation, while the buttons correspond to her continuing dependency. Interestingly, the left hand, which had 6 fingers at 13, now has only 4. The lines on the skirt and the heavily-shaded male figure indicate increasing sexual anxiety.

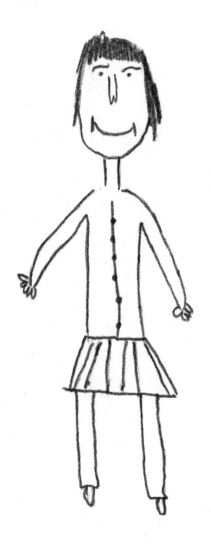

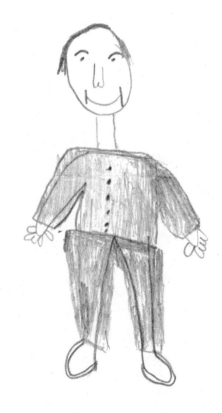

FIGURE 176   FIGURE 177

I.D. *Age 16 & 18* *Female*

This patient came to the clinic for the treatment of allergic rhinitis. Emotional and school difficulties were denied. It is clear from the highly primitive drawings that further psychiatric investigation is warranted.

Drawings: The patient chooses to draw nude figures, males first. The heads of the males are especially primitive, lacking hair, pupils and ears. Noses and mouths are simple gashes. The poorly proportioned outstretched arms with ill-defined hands are totally infantile. The legs pressed together, done with a single line, reflect rigid control over sexual impulses or fear of sexual attack by others. The lack of feet further emphasizes the total dependency and insecurity of this girl.

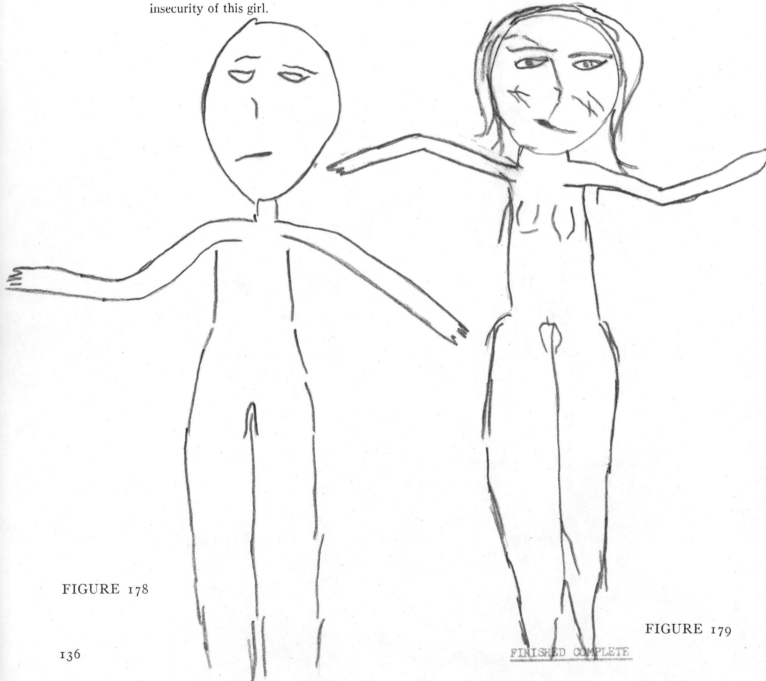

FIGURE 178

FIGURE 179

FINISHED COMPLETE

At 18 the essential character of these drawings remains unchanged, but some maturation has taken place. The beginning descent of the arms is a sign of a lessened "carry me" attitude. Nipples, breasts and genitalia are prominently displayed and the legs are separated. The patient is now more able to accept sexuality. However, the explicit presence of genitalia on such primitive figures in a girl of almost adult years raises serious diagnostic questions.

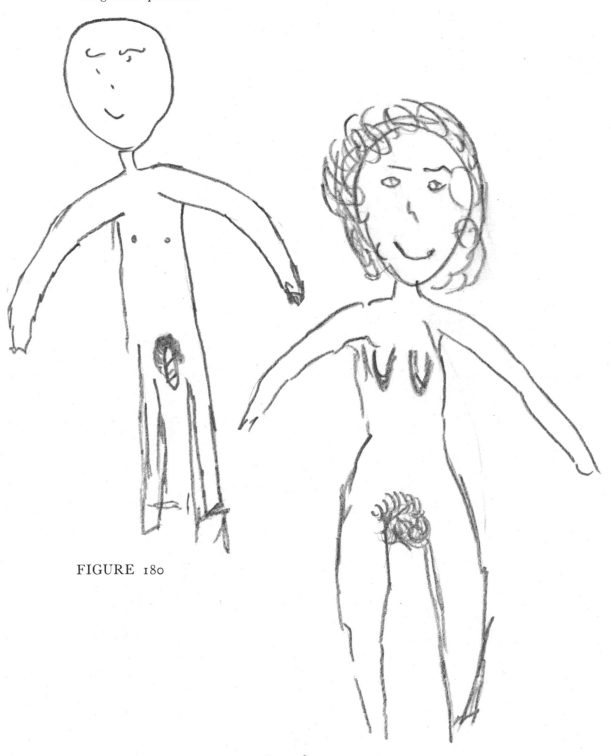

FIGURE 180

FIGURE 181

FIGURES 182, 183

I.E.   *Age 16 & 18*   *Male*

The patient suffers from fatigue and nose bleeds. He has difficulty falling asleep, has few friends and does poorly in school. He smokes marijuana. His major difficulty is with his father, an angry, jealous man. Shortly after his first visit to the clinic, the boy wounded his father with a screwdriver. The hand grenade actually portended this incident (see Chapter IX, *Danger Signals*).

Drawings: These well-done figures demonstrate a partial shift in drive interest from aggressive to sexual within a 2-year period. Cultural determinants are present. The first, not particularly Negro in character, tells a story of rage and destruction. At age 18 the male figure depicted is a powerful nude, virile and impregnable, with an Afro haircut. The clenched fists have taken the place of a hand grenade—in effect, he can take care of himself now.

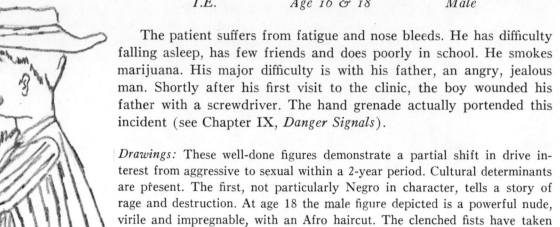

FIGURE 182

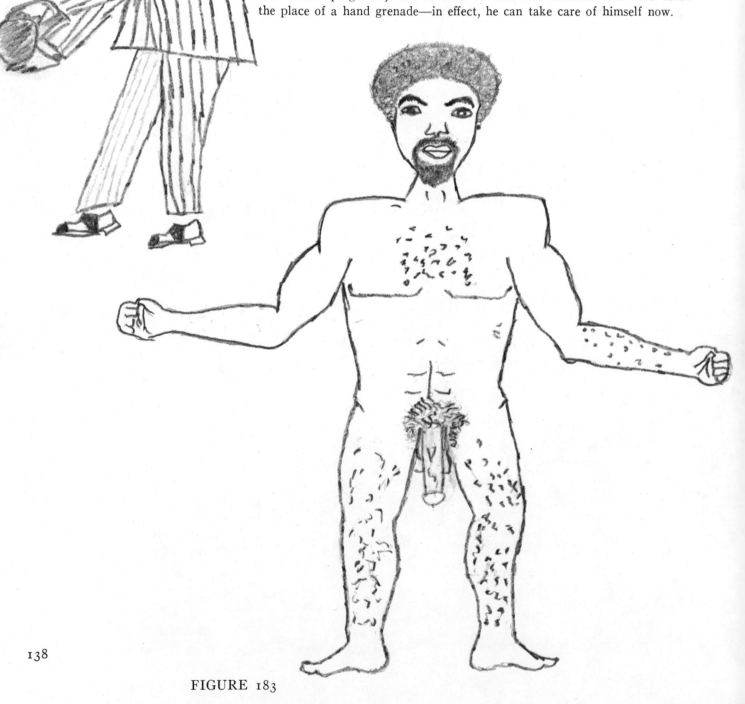

138

FIGURE 183

I.F.   *Age 16 & 18*   *Male*

At 16 this enuretic patient learned that he was a severe diabetic, difficult to control. He became depressed and disinterested in school, dropping out a term before graduation. Always a quiet boy, he withdrew from friends and family. Two years later he had made an excellent adjustment. Accepting his diabetes, learning to live with it, he got himself a job and a renewed sense of pride. His enuresis subsided. He took a high school equivalence examination and began to move out tentatively into the world of peers.

Drawings: At 16, at the height of his depression, he drew a stick figure with 2 dots for eyes. This reflected his almost total decathexis of life. Medically, it was feared that he might commit suicide by neglecting his diabetes (see Chapter IX on *Danger Signals*).

At 18 he draws a total man, albeit somewhat rigid. The hands pointing inward imply somatic concern, realistic in view of his chronic illness. The eyes lack pupils. The twisted mouth is agape and has something in it, perhaps his tongue. The restrictions on his diet may explain the skewed mouth and the wish not to see. The drawings of the female add nothing more to our understanding and are therefore omitted.

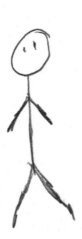

FIGURE 184

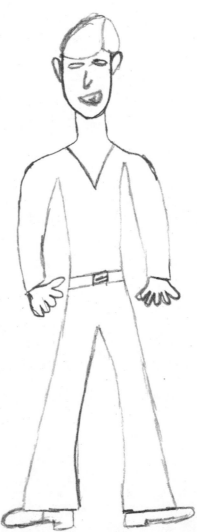

FIGURE 185

I.G. *Age 17 & 19* *Female*

The patient came to the clinic for the treatment of severe obesity. In the first 8 months she lost 21 lbs.; in the next 16 months she gained 77 lbs.

Drawings: These were chosen to demonstrate the static persistence of two pathological findings characteristic of gross immaturity over a 2-year period. Just as she projected little change in her human figure drawings, so did she maintain her obese physical state.

The boy figure done at age 17 (figure 186), stands with arms outstretched in the manner of a young child reaching for succor. There are 6 fingers on the right hand. The patient does not have polydactyly. At 19, although the figures are now larger and a little freer, they still have outstretched arms and 6 fingers! A wide-open mouth has replaced the single smiling line. Denial of the central problem of obesity persists, as do wishes for instant gratification.

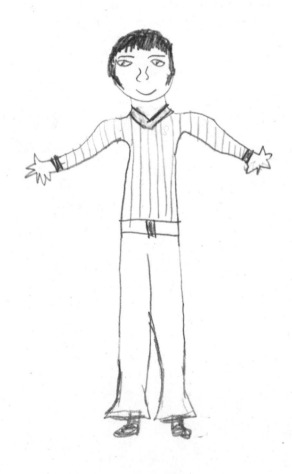

FIGURE 186

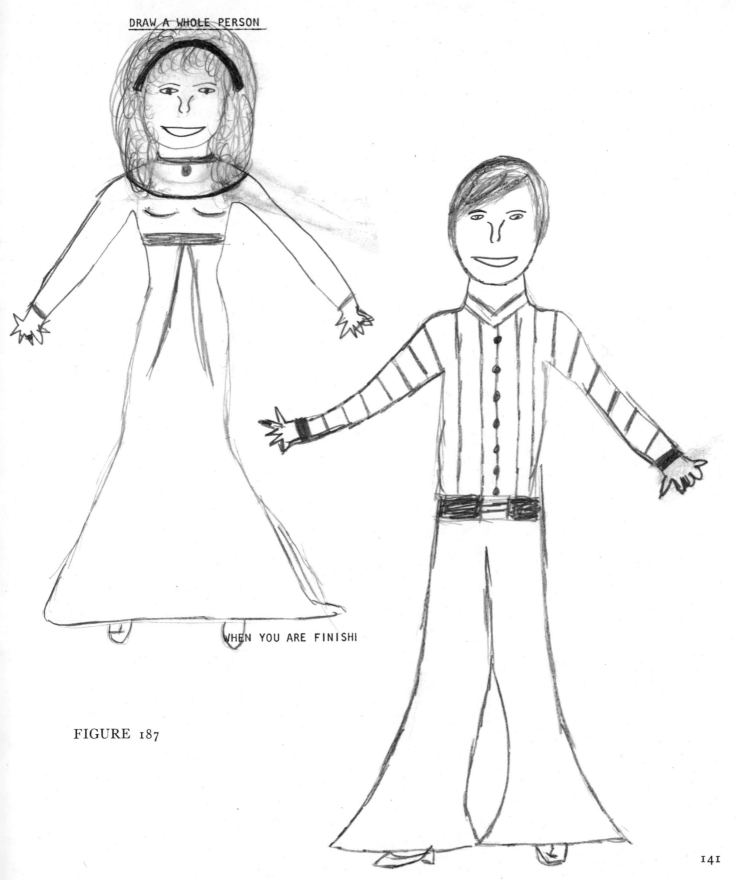

DRAW A WHOLE PERSON

WHEN YOU ARE FINISHI

FIGURE 187

FIGURE 188

141

I.H. *Age 16 & 17½* *Male*

The patient suffers from bronchial asthma. Attacks are often clearly precipitated by emotional factors. He is an anxious boy, unable to express his emotions directly. Psychological testing revealed marked somatization and unconscious hostility, especially toward his mother.

Drawings: They demonstrate a marked degree of regression in a 1½-year period. We do not know the reasons for this, or whether the regression is transient in nature. On the basis of these drawings, the patient's mental health should be more intensively investigated.

The drawings done at 16 show no distinction between male and female. They are lightly drawn with broken lines, indicating anxiety. The general impression is one of immaturity. There is a lack of detail throughout. The limp arms are foreshortened.

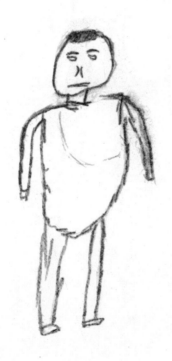

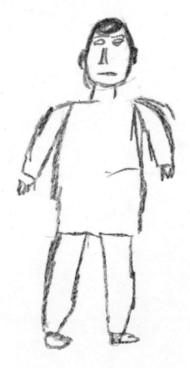

FIGURE 189 FIGURE 190

At 17½ the patient seems to be in severe conflict. He draws and scribbles over his productions time and again. Despite his efforts, he ends up with tiny, immature balloon-type figures. A little more hair distinguishes the primitive female from the male.

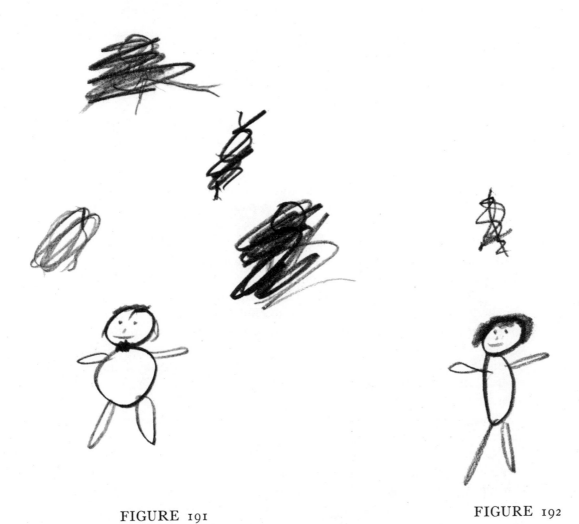

FIGURE 191   FIGURE 192

CHAPTER XI

Conclusion

Our primary interest is the psychology of adolescence. The rapid growth of adolescent medical clinics and in-patient services throughout the country, designed to serve youth from 12 to 19 as *total* human beings, has created new needs. These services are staffed by professional and para-professional personnel trained in different disciplines. Confrontation with the emotional problems of this most turbulent period of life tends to stimulate considerable anxiety in those staff members who have had little exposure to clinical psychiatry. Through conferences, live case presentations and on the spot consultations, it is possible over a period of time to raise the level of psychological sophistication and sensitivity of our staff members and thereby reduce their anxiety to some degree. It is never possible, and perhaps not even desirable, to totally eliminate this anxiety because it serves as a motivational lever to continue the learning process and improve self-mastery in dealing with adolescents.

This book was born in our recognition of the need to find a simple, relatively rapid and understandable tool to alert the non-psychiatric clinician and health and guidance personnel to the possible existence of significant emotional problems or subtle cerebral organic pathology in patients with a wide variety of complaints and behavioral manifestations, often seemingly unrelated to their mental state. In the recently released (July 1971) report on "Stability and Disruption in the Public Schools of New York City" made by Chancellor Harvey B. Scribner's school stability resource team, the comment is made that "Guidance personnel are not diagnosing disruptive children's problems and referrals are not being made to proper agencies." Understanding of the communication inherent in the human figure drawing, its ready availability and relative simplicity can assist counsellors in the first important step: case-finding. Implicit in this concept is the hope of preventive benefits.

It is the first contact with the adolescent that sets the tone for the future clinic-patient, counsellor or doctor-patient relationship. If he is to trust us, cooperate in following recommendations and return when he needs us, we must offer him more than routine medical care or rational advice. We must, above all, relate to him with respect and concern. Never was there a greater need for in-depth understanding of the adolescent than today. Any movement in that direction must bring mutual rewards.

We have found the use of the human figure drawing a highly revealing and useful tool in spotting psychopathology of all varieties. It does not in itself make a diagnosis, but it does ring an alarm bell in the mind of the observer. There are, indeed, patients in whom serious mental symptoms are manifest and yet who draw the human figure within acceptable normal limits. In our series such patients are rare and those whom we investigated have one important thing in common: their pre-adolescent ego was adequately structured. As Brody points out: "The first inside picture which the human individual has of himself is an image of his body." If this image is intact in early childhood, later stresses may not necessarily destroy it, although transient aberrations do appear (see figures 130, 132). For the great majority, disturbances of body image are a central problem at some time during the span of adolescent years. Because of the instability of his ego ideals and his over-dependence on the real or fantasied judgement of his peers, the adolescent is highly vulnerable to anxiety over his body image. The human figure drawing, used as a projective device, tells us much about the individual's current concept of himself. This concept is a composite of his actual physical appearance and his conscious and unconscious internalized self-representation. The more disturbed the adolescent, the less role reality or a wished-for idealization plays in the portrait that he produces. The adolescent is notably intolerant and ashamed of even the mildest physical defects in himself, exaggerating their effect on others and blaming these defects for all sorts of behavioral inadequacies and affective disturbances.

Our study of human figure drawings produced by a random population of adolescents in a general hospital medical clinic and in-patient service, as well as a collection from a junior high school and freshman college class, leads us to a number of observations more specifically applicable to this age group. Most striking is the enormous range in the maturity levels in a 7-year age span. Among the normal, maturation develops more or less in harmony with chronological advancement, allowing for some transient deviations and regressions due to inevitable stress situations. Hero stereotypes, figures in motion and environmental embellishments are far less common in adolescence than in the younger child. What we do see, much more commonly than we anticipated, are adolescents even as old as 19 drawing the human figure at levels expected of normal children under the age of 12 (Goodenough scale). These drawings are often at variance with the clinical impression conveyed by an intelligent, physically mature youth with good, but sometimes misleading verbal skills. In Chapter III on *Personality Traits,* we demonstrated a number of drawings of this type of immature and inadequate self-representation. Some look like puppets, waiting to be manipulated by others (figure 17). In our follow-up study, these same traits tend to persist, even when there is refinement in drawing technique. It is not possible for us to state with certainty whether current methods of upbringing, or educational and cultural factors, have played a role in producing widespread self-concepts of immaturity and dependency. Further research in this area on a more widespread scale, buttressed with statistics and done over a decade, might help to clarify this most significant question, about which there has been so much speculation. In our patient population, predominantly middle class, we see very little in the drawings that distinguishes the black from the white youth. The Afro hair-do is popularly drawn, but on occasion it is offered by a white adolescent. In only one instance was the skin colored in black by a 12-year-old Negro girl (figure 4). A few of the drawings done by black male patients show strongly aggressive fantasies, but many are passive and immature. There is no striking statistical difference in our sample, reenforcing the premise that socio-economic factors, more than racial, determine the adolescent's self-image. There are signs, however, that in the past two years the older black adolescent has begun to project an image of growing racial pride.

In organic brain damage and psychosis one expects to see the stigmata of developmental lag and deviations. These expectations are fulfilled in the illustrations offered in Chapters VI and VIII. In organicity there are specific signs such as a high number of omissions, disproportions, displacements, etc., which change little or not at all with age. One cannot determine anything especially characteristic of adolescence in the neurologically damaged. In psychosis the picture is one of great variety, fluidity, confusion, and bizarreness. In these drawings the severity of the illness, the degree of regression or fixation, and the nature of the fantasy life are the determinants of the projected material. If the fantasies of the patient are focused on adolescent problems, as they often are, the human figure drawings are more age-specific. Follow-up drawings mirror the life history, showing progression, regression or a relatively static state, never fully identical with the past.

Physical illness, even of minor degree, causes an exceptionally severe narcissistic blow to adolescents. It provokes regression at a time of life particularly susceptible to backwards movement, for reasons explained in Chapter II on *Parameters of Normalcy*. Most commonly, the adolescent deals with the anxiety provoked by illness with the unconscious mechanism of denial. In the drawings this is demonstrated by the removal of the affected part of the body. This is not a universal mode of response. Sometimes the affected region is distorted or the illness exaggerated. For example, there are illustrations showing featureless faces (figure 56) and others showing huge pimples (figure 45) in cases of juvenile acne. Adolescents are especially disturbed by any illness that affects their physical appearance, suffering intense shame, sometimes without basis in reality. Obesity, one of the most common afflictions of this age period, does not appear in a single one of the drawings of patients with this condition. Instead, an idealized wished-for body is often presented. In cases of life-threatening illness, one is struck by a number of drawings of dehumanized armatures (figures 56, 59). The patient appears to have decathected his body and is ready for the surgeon's knife or even death, and hopes to avoid the terror and pain by not feeling.

The drawings that express the evolution of sexual identity in adolescence and problems arising from it tell the most compelling story of all. In them we see the striking changes that normally take place between ages 12 and 19. The wishes, guilt, fears, preoccupation and oedipal conflicts are all demonstrated. Nude figures with explicit genitalia seem to appear with greater frequency in this age group than in a random adult population (Machover).

Many of the drawings that indicate the probable presence of a neurotic conflict have a depressed or anxious quality that elicits empathic responses in the adult observer. Memories of forgotten adolescent pain and struggle are vaguely stirred up. A sense of anomie is illustrated in figure 109. In general, the level of developmental maturity in these drawings is high, as contrasted with those which illustrate psychosis and organicity.

147

In Chapter IX on *Danger Signals,* we illustrate the predictive possibility of an occasional drawing demonstrating strong aggressive impulses directed against the self or others. If the history or interview even minimally supports the possibility of a harmful act, these drawings should be taken seriously. Such patients deserve more intense investigation.

In this study we have attempted to bring to your attention the value of the simple human figure drawing as a projective diagnostic tool during the fluid years of adolescence. Our material has been gathered from a non-psychiatric population and emphasizes the frequency of undetected and untreated emotional problems among our youth. Understanding these drawings has been invaluable and richly rewarding to us. It is our hope that the reader will share our enthusiasm.

References

BENDER, L.: *A Visual Motor Gestalt Test and Its Clinical Use*. The American Orthopsychiatric Association Research Monograph, No. 3, 1938

BENDER, L.: The Drawing of a Man in Chronic Encephalitis in Children. *J. Nerv. Mental Dis.*, 41: 277-286, 1960.

BENDER, L.: Some Art Work of Emotionally Disturbed Boys at Puberty, *J. Hillside Hospital*, V. XVII, No. 4: 349-361, Oct. 1968.

BLOS, P.: *On Adolescence: A Psychoanalytic Interpretation*. New York: Free Press, 1962.

BRODY, S.: *Patterns of Mothering*. New York: International Univ. Press, 1966.

BUCK, J. N.: The H-T-P Technique: A Qualitative and Quantitative Scoring Manuel, *J. Clin. Psychol. J. Clin. Psychol.*, 4: 317-396, 1948.

BURNS, R. C. and KAUFMAN, S. H.: *Kinetic Family Drawings*. New York: Brunner/Mazel, 1970.

DI LEO, J.: *Young Children and Their Drawings*. New York: Brunner/Mazel, 1970.

ELKIND, D. and SCOTT, L.: Studies in Perceptual Development, I. The Decentering of Perception. *Child Devel.* 33: 619-631.

FEINSTEIN, S., GIOVACCHINI, P. and MILLER, A., Editors: *Adolescent Psychiatry*, Vol. 1. Developmental & Clinical Studies, 1970.

FREUD, A.: Technique of Child Analysis. *Nerv. & Ment. Diseases Monograph*, No. 48: 1928.

GOODENOUGH, F. L.: *Measurement of Intelligence by Drawings*. New York: Harcourt, Brace & World, Inc. 1926.

HAMIS, D. B.: *Children's Drawings as Measures of Intellect and Maturity*. New York: Harcourt, Brace & World, Inc., 1963.

HAMMER, E. F.: *The Clinical Application of Projective Drawings*. Springfield, Ill.: Charles C Thomas, 1958.

JOLLES, I.: *A Catalogue for the Qualitative Interpretation of the H-T-P*. Beverly Hills, Calif.: Western Psychological Services, 1952.

KOPPITZ, E. M.: *Psychological Evaluation of Children's Human Figure Drawings*. New York: Grune and Stratton, 1968.

MACHOVER, K.: *Personality Projection in the Drawing of the Human Figure*. Springfield, Ill.: Charles C Thomas, 1949.

PHELAN, H. M.: The Incidence and Possible Significance of the Drawing of Female Figures by Sixth Grade Boys in Response to the Draw a Person Test. *Psychiat. Quart.*, 38: 488-503, 1964.

SCHILDER, P.: *Image and Appearance of the Human Body*. New York: International Univ. Press, 1935.

SCHILDKROUT, M. and SHENKER, I. R.: Headaches and Abdominal Pains in the Adolescent. *Clinical Pediatrics* 7: 55-58, 1968.

SCHILDKROUT, M.: The Pediatrician and the Child Psychiatrist. *J. Hillside Hospital*, Vol. XIV No. 3. 152-159. July, 1965.

SCHUYTEN, M. C.: De Oorsprokelijke Vertges der Antwerpsche School Kindern, *Pead. Jaarb*, 5, 1-87, 1904.

SIMON, M.: L'Imagination dans la Folie: Etude sur les Dessins, Plans, Descriptions, et Costumes des Aliénés, *Ann. Medico Psychol.*, 16: 358-390, 1876.

Index